THE COMPLETE KETO DIET AFTER 60

By Amelia Sanchez

Table of Contents

Before you start reading, scan this QR Code to get all bonus content!

INTRODUCTION

Welcome aboard, dear reader! This is the start of something special—a journey tailored for the fabulous women navigating the vibrant tapestry of life beyond 60. In the chapters that follow, we're delving into the world of the ketogenic (keto) diet, a thoughtful exploration designed to bring forth better health, vitality, and a renewed zest for life.

Unveiling the Essence of Keto

Ever wondered about the buzz around the keto diet? Well, it's like discovering a secret passage to wellness. Together we will unravel the history and principles behind keto—no complex jargon, just a friendly guide into why keto might be your ticket to feeling fantastic. Our bodies are incredible storytellers, especially as we gracefully age. In this book, we're having a heart-to-heart about those changes. Think of it as a roadmap to understanding the subtle shifts in hormones, metabolism, and overall well-being that come with the territory of being a fantastic woman in her 60s.

Personal Solutions

Weight, metabolism, staying peppy—real concerns, right? But worry not, this book is like a trusted friend offering solutions. It's about tailoring the keto lifestyle to fit your groove—a holistic approach to wellness that resonates with your unique journey beyond 60. As you flip through these pages, imagine it as an elegant invitation. This isn't just about diets; it's a rendezvous with a healthier, more vibrant version of you. Keto isn't a rigid rulebook; it's a gentle guide to feeling fantastic and embracing the richness of life beyond 60.

So, here's to the journey—a voyage into keto, wellness, and the vibrant chapters that lie ahead.

The intended readership for "Keto Diet for Women Over 60" comprises women who are 60 years of age or older, seeking to improve their health, manage their weight, and lead a more active and fulfilling life through the adoption of the ketogenic (keto) diet. This specific audience possesses distinctive characteristics, challenges, and aspirations, which are elucidated below:

CHAPTER 1: INTRODUCTION TO THE KETO DIET

Welcome to a transformative journey into the world of the ketogenic (keto) diet—a path that holds incredible promise for revitalizing your health and well-being. In this opening chapter, we'll demystify the keto approach, making it not just a dietary choice but a companion in your pursuit of a healthier and more vibrant life beyond 60.

Unraveling Keto: What's It All About?

Embarking on the journey of the ketogenic (keto) diet is akin to stepping into a realm where science, nutrition, and transformative results converge. This isn't a passing trend but rather a lifestyle that draws its essence from a deep understanding of our bodies and how they interact with the food we consume. Let's delve into the intricacies of keto, exploring why it transcends the realm of mere dieting to become a way of life.

The Science Behind Keto

At its core, keto is a metabolic marvel grounded in scientific principles. To grasp its essence, we need to venture into the realm of macronutrients—those essential components that make up our daily diet. While traditional diets often revolve around calorie counting, keto takes a different route, focusing on the quality and composition of those calories.

A Macro View: Redefining Nutrient Intake

In the world of keto, macronutrients take center stage, and there are three main players: fats, proteins, and carbohydrates. Here's the twist—while carbs have been the go-to energy source for our bodies, keto flips the script. By significantly reducing carbohydrate intake and replacing it with healthy fats, we prompt a remarkable shift in how our bodies derive and utilize energy.

The Ketosis Conundrum

Now, let's talk about the star of the show: ketosis. This isn't a mysterious state; it's a metabolic process where the body, deprived of its usual carb fuel, starts burning stored fats for energy. It's like activating an internal power plant that torches fat reserves, leading to weight loss and, more importantly, a consistent and sustained energy source.

Redefining Our Relationship with Food

Keto isn't just a list of do's and don'ts; it's a profound shift in our approach to eating. It invites us to reconsider the very nature of our relationship with food. Instead of viewing food as a mere source of calories, keto encourages us to see it as a tool for nourishment, fuel, and overall well-being.

Beyond Calorie Counting

In a world fixated on calorie reduction, keto stands out by emphasizing the quality of calories over sheer quantity. It's not just about eating less; it's about eating right. By embracing healthy fats and moderating protein intake, we find ourselves satiated and energized without the need to constantly monitor calorie intake.

Energy Stability: The Keto Advantage

One of the standout features of keto is its ability to provide a stable and sustained energy source. Unlike the energy spikes and crashes often associated with high-carb diets, keto offers a more consistent fuel supply. It's like trading the flickering flame of a candle for the steady glow of a lantern, providing a reliable source of energy throughout the day.

Keto as a Lifestyle

Here's the real magic of keto—it's not a crash diet or a temporary fix. It's a lifestyle, a way of approaching nutrition that can be sustained over the long haul. This isn't about quick fixes; it's about cultivating a relationship with food that nurtures your body and supports your health journey.

The Freedom of Food Choices

Contrary to restrictive diets, keto opens up a world of delicious possibilities. Avocado, nuts, olive oil— these become not just allowed but encouraged. Keto isn't about deprivation; it's about embracing a diverse and satisfying range of foods while staying true to the fundamental principles that make it work.

A Shift in Mindset

Perhaps the most transformative aspect of keto is the shift in mindset it encourages. It's about breaking free from the conventional narrative of dieting as a constant struggle. With keto, food becomes a source of empowerment, a tool for achieving your health and wellness goals.

So, as we embark on this journey into the heart of keto, remember—it's not just a diet; it's a profound redefinition of how we nourish our bodies, energize our lives, and embrace a lifestyle that stands the test of time. Get ready for a transformation that goes beyond the plate!

Origins and Evolution of Keto

Understanding the keto diet isn't just about knowing what to eat; it's about appreciating where this transformative lifestyle originated and how it has evolved over time. So, buckle up for a historical journey that begins in the 1920s, weaving through scientific breakthroughs, medical applications, and the revelation of keto's multifaceted potential.

A Glimpse Into the Roaring Twenties

Picture a world where flapper dresses, jazz music, and Model Ts dominated the scene. It's the 1920s, and amidst this cultural upheaval, a medical breakthrough quietly emerges. Dr. Russell Wilder, a Mayo Clinic physician, introduces the ketogenic diet as a therapeutic approach for epilepsy. Epilepsy, a condition marked by recurrent seizures, posed a considerable challenge for medical professionals at the time. Dr. Wilder's ketogenic diet, which emphasized high-fat, low-carbohydrate, and adequate protein intake, offered a novel solution. The idea was to induce a state of ketosis, altering the brain's energy metabolism and reducing seizure activity.

From Medical Niche to Mainstream Spotlight

As the decades unfolded, the ketogenic diet remained primarily within the realm of epilepsy treatment. However, it wasn't long before its potential reached beyond seizure control. Researchers and medical professionals began to explore its applications in diverse areas, unveiling a more comprehensive understanding of the profound impact keto could have on our health. One of the first areas to capture attention was weight management. In the 1960s, Dr. Atkins introduced a lowcarbohydrate diet that shared striking similarities with the ketogenic approach. This sparked a renewed interest in the diet's potential beyond epilepsy, laying the groundwork for its evolution into a weight-loss tool.

Metabolic Resonance

The 1980s witnessed a surge in scientific inquiry into metabolic health. Researchers began recognizing the role of insulin and glucose in the development of metabolic disorders. The ketogenic diet, with its ability to modulate insulin and glucose levels, emerged as a promising strategy for addressing metabolic issues such as insulin resistance and type 2 diabetes. Fast forward to the present day, and keto has stepped into the mainstream spotlight, no longer confined to medical journals. It has become a dynamic and versatile lifestyle embraced by individuals seeking not just weight loss but a holistic approach to health.

A Tool for Weight Management

The keto diet's efficacy in weight management has been extensively studied and acknowledged. Its ability to tap into fat stores for energy, coupled with the satiating effect of fats, has made it a go-to choice for those looking to shed excess pounds and maintain a healthy weight. Beyond weight, keto's influence on metabolic health continues to captivate researchers. The diet's impact on insulin sensitivity, blood sugar regulation, and lipid profiles showcases its potential as a preventive and therapeutic tool against metabolic disorders.

Cognitive Clarity

Recent research has also illuminated keto's impact on cognitive function. The diet's potential neuroprotective effects and its application in conditions like Alzheimer's disease have opened new avenues for exploration in the realm of brain health. In tracing the origins and evolution of the ketogenic diet, we witness a journey that transcends medical applications, stepping into the realms of weight management, metabolic health, and cognitive well-being. Today, keto stands not only as a historical testament but as a contemporary lifestyle choice—a tool with the power to transform lives and redefine our relationship with health.

So, as we navigate the keto landscape in this guide, remember that its roots run deep, connecting the scientific breakthroughs of the past to the diverse health benefits we explore today.

Breaking Down the Basics

Embarking on the keto journey is like stepping onto a stage where your body becomes the lead performer in a metabolic symphony. To truly appreciate this performance, let's unravel the basics of keto—a graceful dance between macronutrients, energy sources, and a transformative state known as ketosis.

The Macronutrient Ballet

Keto's first move involves a shift in our macronutrient consumption—those essential nutrients our bodies need in larger quantities. Imagine macronutrients as the principal dancers in our dietary ballet: fats, proteins, and carbohydrates. In the standard dietary routine, carbohydrates take center stage. They are our body's preferred source of energy, quickly converted into glucose for immediate use. But in the keto ballet, carbohydrates gracefully take a step back. By significantly reducing their presence, we usher in a new era of energy production.

The Rise of Healthy Fats

Enter healthy fats—the unsung heroes of the keto narrative. As carbohydrates bow out, fats take the lead, becoming the primary source of energy. This shift encourages the body to tap into its fat stores, initiating a process that lies at the heart of the keto magic—entering the state of ketosis. While fats shine as the main attraction, proteins play a supporting role. Adequate protein intake is essential to maintain muscle mass and support various bodily functions. It's all about finding the delicate balance between fats, proteins, and carbs to create a macronutrient masterpiece.

The Keto Magic: Entering Ketosis

Now, let's talk about the star of the show—ketosis. It's not a mysterious realm but rather a metabolic state where the body's primary energy source shifts from glucose to ketones, which are produced from fat breakdown. Here's how this enchanting process unfolds: With reduced carbohydrate intake, the body exhausts its glucose reserves, prompting a metabolic switch. Carbohydrates, which once fueled our energy, step back, creating an opportunity for a more sustainable and efficient source to take the spotlight.

Fats Take Center Stage

As carbs gracefully bow out, fats become the headliners. Our bodies, now fueled by fatty acids, initiate the breakdown of fat stores into ketones—a process that not only provides a consistent energy supply but also prompts the efficient burning of stored fat. Ketones, the byproduct of fat metabolism, become the maestros of this metabolic symphony. These molecules circulate in the bloodstream, serving as an alternative energy source for organs, including the brain. It's a harmonious dance between fats, ketones, and metabolic efficiency. Now, this may sound like a complex orchestration, but fear not! The beauty of keto lies in its simplicity. It's not about intricate calculations or obscure scientific principles; it's about understanding the basics of a dietary shift that transforms your body's energy dynamics.

Practical Insight: Your Body, the Fat Burner

In essence, keto turns your body into a highly efficient fat-burning machine. By reducing carbs and upping healthy fats, you create an environment where stored fat becomes the primary fuel. It's a metabolic adaptation that not only aids in weight management but also offers a steady, reliable source of energy throughout your day. In the upcoming chapters, we'll break down these concepts further, providing practical insights into meal planning, food choices, and the day-to-day application of keto principles. Consider this your backstage pass to the keto symphony, where the magic unfolds in a way that's easy to grasp and incorporate into your lifestyle. So, as we lift the curtain on the basics of keto, get ready to embrace the transformative melody of macronutrients, energy efficiency, and the symphony of ketosis. The stage is set, and the keto journey awaits!

The Promise for Women Over 60

As we set sail into the realm of the ketogenic (keto) diet, a beacon of curiosity may arise: "Why keto, especially for the incredible women navigating their way through the vibrant tapestry of their 60s?" This, my dear reader, is a question that unravels the magic inherent in the keto journey—a journey meticulously tailored to address the distinctive health considerations of this pivotal life stage.

Decoding the Enigma: Why Keto for Women in Their 60s?

Picture this: a symphony of hormones, metabolic nuances, and decades of life experiences. In the grand orchestra of a woman's body after 60, metabolic changes take center stage. Here's where keto dons its tailored elegance, offering a strategic approach to navigate the intricate dance of insulin, glucose, and the quest for a stable, resilient metabolism.

Yes, keto holds promise for weight management, but it's not a singular melody; it's part of a harmonious composition. As women gracefully age, the challenge of maintaining a healthy weight becomes more nuanced. Keto steps in not just as a weight-loss strategy but as a holistic symphony, considering factors like muscle preservation, energy stability, and the preservation of overall well-being.

In the life score beyond 60, bone health takes on added significance. Keto, with its emphasis on nutrient-dense foods, contributes to the preservation of bone density. The diet becomes a melodic note in the ongoing composition of supporting skeletal strength and resilience. For women over 60 seeking an enduring vitality, keto emerges as a tune that plays in harmony with the rhythms of daily life.

The Holistic Score: It's Beyond Weight Loss

Now, let's address the core of the melody. The keto diet for women over 60 is not a one-dimensional tune solely focused on shedding pounds. It's a holistic composition, a tailored score that harmonizes with the unique needs and aspirations of this life stage.

In the grand performance of life, cognitive health takes a starring role. Keto, with its potential neuroprotective effects, becomes a nourishing note in supporting brain health. The diet is not just about numbers on a scale; it's about sustaining mental clarity, memory, and overall cognitive well-being. Hormones, the conductors of the body's intricate orchestra, undergo shifts as women age. Keto steps in as a balancing act, influencing hormonal stability. From insulin sensitivity to estrogen levels, the diet becomes a supportive melody in navigating the hormonal changes that accompany this life stage.

Keto, with its potential mood-stabilizing effects, becomes a note that resonates with the emotional well-being of women over 60. It's about fostering a positive relationship with food, body, and self.

The Essence of Keto: A Tailored Serenade

In essence, keto for women over 60 is not just a diet; it's a tailored serenade—a composition that addresses the multifaceted dimensions of health and well-being. It's a recognition that each woman's journey is unique, and the keto diet becomes a personalized melody that enhances the vibrancy of life beyond 60.

So, as we navigate the promise of keto, envision it not as a mere diet but as a resonant tune—an eloquent piece crafted to elevate, support, and celebrate the remarkable journey of women beyond 60. The stage is set, the orchestra is tuned, and the promise of keto unfolds in a symphony of well-being.

The Physiology of Change: A Deep Dive into the Symphony of Aging

As we gracefully embrace the passage of time, our bodies embark on a profound journey of transformation. This chapter unfolds as a narrative, a voyage into the intricate symphony of physiological changes that accompanies the tapestry of aging. Let's take an extensive exploration, delving into the nuances of how these shifts play out, conducting a harmonious examination of metabolism, hormonal dynamics, and the overarching canvas of health. It is within this intricate understanding that we discover the compelling reasons why the keto diet emerges as a transformative force for women navigating the splendid realm of their 60s.

The Metabolic Ballet: A Refined Choreography

Picture metabolism as a ballet dancer, gracefully adapting to the changing tempo of life. With age, the metabolic rate encounters subtle variations. It's not a sudden crescendo but a gradual modulation—a nuanced shift that can impact how our bodies process and utilize energy. Enter keto as a choreographer, offering a strategic routine that aligns with the evolving rhythms of metabolic grace.

Insulin, the conductor of our body's glucose orchestra, experiences changes in sensitivity over time. This delicate dance between insulin and glucose becomes more intricate with each passing year. Keto steps onto the stage, guiding this pas de deux with its focus on low-carbohydrate intake, potentially enhancing insulin sensitivity and supporting a balanced glycemic performance.

Hormonal Harmony: A Symphony of Change

In the grand symphony of hormonal changes, estrogen takes a front-row seat. As women traverse through their 60s, estrogen levels experience a gradual ebb and flow. Keto enters as a melodic note, potentially influencing hormonal stability and offering a supportive refrain amidst the hormonal shifts that accompany this life stage.

The thyroid, the conductor orchestrating metabolism, undergoes its own modulation. Aging introduces subtle variations in thyroid function, impacting the overall tempo of metabolic processes. Keto, with its potential influence on metabolism, steps in as a complementary melody, working in tandem with the thyroid's natural rhythm.

The Canvas of Overall Health: Painting with Precision

Inflammation, a background note in the symphony of health, may undergo shifts as we age. Chronic inflammation, often associated with aging, can influence various aspects of well-being. Keto, with its potential anti-inflammatory effects, becomes an artist's brush, delicately painting a canvas of health with strokes of precision and care.

The subtle undertone of oxidative stress emerges as another theme in the aging symphony. Our bodies, exposed to the passage of time, may encounter increased oxidative stress. Keto, with its focus on antioxidant-rich foods, introduces a counterpoint—a gentle undertone that seeks to balance the intricacies of oxidative stress.

A Synthesis of Understanding: Why Keto?

In understanding these physiological shifts, we unlock the secrets of why the keto diet stands as a game-changer for women in their 60s. It's not just about shedding light on the changes but orchestrating a response that aligns with the evolving needs of the body. Keto becomes a tailored composition, resonating with the cadence of metabolic, hormonal, and overall health transformations.

So, as we immerse ourselves in the physiology of change, envision it as a masterful symphony—the aging body as the orchestra, and keto as the conductor guiding each instrument with precision and expertise. The curtain rises on a performance where health, well-being, and the grace of aging unite in a captivating composition.

NavigatingCommon Concerns: A Comprehensive VoyageThrough Keto's Landscape of Wellness

Embarking on a new dietary journey is akin to setting sail on uncharted waters, filled with anticipation, curiosity, and yes, a fair share of questions and concerns. For the remarkable women in their 60s stepping into the world of keto, these concerns span a spectrum, from the intricacies of weight management to the nuances of sustaining energy levels. In this chapter, we don't merely acknowledge these common worries; we confront them head-on, unfurling a detailed map that provides not only insights but practical solutions to ensure a seamless transition into the captivating realm of keto.

Weight Management: Beyond the Numbers

As the years gracefully unfold, weight management becomes a nuanced ballet. For women in their 60s, the concern isn't merely about shedding pounds; it's about navigating the intricate dance between metabolism, hormonal changes, and muscle preservation. Keto, with its focus on preserving lean muscle mass and supporting metabolism, becomes a guiding partner in this weight management journey.

Keto, often celebrated for its weight-loss benefits, is not about swift, unsustainable results. It's a slow waltz, emphasizing sustainable weight loss that aligns with the natural rhythms of the body. By addressing concerns about the pace and longevity of weight loss, we unveil the enduring beauty of keto's contribution to a healthier and more vibrant you.

Energy Levels: Sustaining the Vital Rhythm

Energy, the life force that propels us through each day, takes center stage. In the world of keto, the concern shifts from fleeting energy spikes to the quest for a sustained, reliable energy source. By elucidating the principles of ketones as a steady fuel supply, we demystify the common worry of fluctuating energy levels, revealing how keto can become the conductor of a consistent vitality symphony.

Addressing concerns about energy often involves debunking the myth that carbohydrates are the sole providers of sustained vitality. Keto challenges this notion, introducing the concept of becoming metabolically flexible—shifting from a carbdependent to a fat-adapted energy system. It's a paradigm shift that reshapes the narrative around energy concerns, offering a pathway to enduring vitality.

The Psychological Landscape: Embracing Change

Transitioning into a new dietary lifestyle can evoke psychological shifts. Concerns about adaptability, cravings, and the emotional landscape of change come to the forefront. By delving into the psychology of dietary transformation, we not only acknowledge these concerns but provide strategies to foster psychological resilience, ensuring that the journey into keto becomes an empowering narrative rather than a source of stress.

Navigating concerns is rarely a solo endeavor. Recognizing the importance of support systems—be it from family, friends, or the broader keto community—we shed light on the significance of encouragement, shared experiences, and the emotional scaffolding that can make the transition into keto not just manageable but enriching.

A Call to Adventure: The Promise of Keto Unveiled

As we navigate through the common concerns that often accompany the onset of a keto journey, envision it not as an obstacle course but as a carefully charted adventure. This is an exploration of renewed vitality, improved health, and the unveiling of a more vibrant version of yourself. So, buckle up, dear reader, for this enlightening exploration of the keto diet—a voyage that promises not only a destination of well-being but a transformative journey that reshapes the narrative of health in your 60s.

CHAPTER 2: NAVIGATING HEALTH CONSIDERATIONS FOR WOMEN OVER n60

In the enchanting realm of a woman's life beyond 60, health becomes a cherished companion, and the journey takes on unique nuances. This chapter is a guided exploration through the distinctive health challenges, common concerns, and the tailored embrace of the keto diet for women navigating this vibrant life stage.

The Unique Health Challenges

As the years gracefully unfold, metabolic changes gracefully waltz into the forefront. The once familiar rhythms of energy metabolism shift, influenced by the passage of time and hormonal intricacies. These metabolic marvels aren't hurdles but rather a melodic transition. In the grand orchestration of aging, the keto diet emerges as a harmonious partner, offering a tailored approach to navigate these metabolic nuances.

Weight management for women over 60 transcends the simplistic gaze of the scale. Hormonal fluctuations, muscle preservation, and the evolving metabolic rate dance together in a nuanced ballet. Keto steps onto this stage not as a strict director but as a guiding dance partner. We unravel the layers of weight concerns, illustrating how keto becomes an ally in the pursuit of sustainable weight management, preserving vitality along the way. In the intricate ballet of aging, bone health takes on a leading role. The challenges of maintaining bone density and strength unfold, influenced by both the natural aging process and hormonal shifts. Keto joins this ballet as a choreographer, outlining a nutritional routine that supports and nurtures bone health. It's not just about preserving bones; it's about crafting a symphony of strength and resilience.

Addressing Common Concerns

Metabolism, often misunderstood and underestimated, undergoes changes that beckon understanding. We decode the metabolic shifts with a keto lens, exploring how the diet aligns seamlessly with the evolving needs of the body. From metabolic rate variations to the role of ketones in stabilizing energy, keto's perspective on metabolism becomes a beacon for women navigating the intricacies of their metabolic journey.

Weight management becomes a holistic dance, a choreography of health that extends beyond numerical values. Keto enters this dance not as a strict regimen but as a partner in preserving lean muscle mass, supporting metabolism, and fostering sustainable weight loss. The narrative shifts from rapid results to a steady waltz, embracing the enduring beauty of keto's contribution to a healthier weight and enhanced vitality.

The blueprint for robust bone health unfolds as we delve into the impact of hormonal changes and age on skeletal strength. Keto becomes a vital note in this symphony, emphasizing nutrient-dense foods that contribute to bone density. It's a nutritional approach that transcends the surface, becoming a guiding melody for preserving and nurturing skeletal well-being.

Crafting a Keto Strategy

In this segment, we explore the art of personalization within the realm of the ketogenic diet. There are no generic formulas; instead, we embark on a journey of crafting a keto strategy that aligns with individual preferences, health needs, and the unique composition of each woman's body. It's about tailoring keto, not as a rigid doctrine but as a fluid and personalized composition. This isn't a theoretical exploration but a hands-on guide to integrating keto principles into the everyday lives of women over 60. Practical solutions unfold— from meal planning that caters to metabolic shifts to incorporating bone-nourishing foods into the keto repertoire. It's a bridge between theory and practice, ensuring that keto isn't an abstract concept but a lived experience enriched with vitality.

As we conclude this chapter, envision it as a guiding light illuminating the path forward. The health considerations, concerns, and solutions presented here are not merely information—they are beacons guiding women over 60 toward a holistic and empowered approach to health. The keto diet, tailored to their unique needs, stands as a transformative ally on this journey, promising not just adaptation but flourishing vitality in the chapters that lie ahead.

CHAPTER 3: GETTING STARTEDWITH KETO: A PRACTICAL GUIDE TO

EMBARKING ON THE JOURNEY

Embarking on a keto journey requires a thoughtful and systematic approach. This chapter provides concrete step-by-step guidance on initiating a keto diet, underscores the crucial role of consulting with a healthcare professional, and offers practical tips for setting realistic goals and expectations.

1. Understanding the Basics: Initiating Your Keto Journey

a. Grasping the Fundamentals

Before diving into the keto lifestyle, it's essential to understand the fundamental principles. This includes comprehending the macronutrient breakdown—where fats take precedence, carbohydrates are minimized, and a moderate amount of protein is incorporated. Readers will gain insights into the primary mechanism behind ketosis, where the body transitions from burning carbohydrates for fuel to utilizing fat.

1. Carbohydrate Depletion:

- When we consume carbohydrates, our body breaks them down into glucose, a primary source of energy.
- In a traditional diet rich in carbs, our cells rely on glucose as the main fuel to power various physiological functions.

2. Initiating Ketosis through Carb Restriction:

- The ketogenic journey begins with a deliberate reduction in carbohydrate intake.
- As carb intake decreases, the body's glycogen stores, a storage form of glucose, start depleting.

3. Transition to Fat Metabolism:

- In the absence of sufficient carbohydrates, the body shifts its energy production strategy.
- Fatty acids, derived from dietary fats and stored body fat, become the alternative fuel source.

4. Formation of Ketone Bodies:

- As fats undergo a process called beta-oxidation, ketone bodies are produced in the liver.
- Ketones, including acetoacetate, beta-hydroxybutyrate, and acetone, become the new energy substrates.

5. Ketones as Alternative Fuel:

- Ketones can cross the blood-brain barrier, providing a crucial energy source for the brain.

- Major tissues, including muscles, heart, and other organs, adapt to using ketones for energy in the absence of glucose.

6. Achieving Nutritional Ketosis:

- The state where ketone levels in the blood are elevated is termed nutritional ketosis.
- Nutritional ketosis signifies that the body has successfully transitioned from relying on carbohydrates to primarily utilizing fats and ketones for energy.

Key Takeaways:

- *Carbohydrate Depletion Initiates the Process:* The reduction in carbohydrate intake serves as the catalyst, signaling the body to seek alternative energy sources.
- *Fats Become the Primary Fuel:* With lowered glucose availability, the body prioritizes fats as the primary fuel substrate.
- *Ketone Bodies Bridge the Gap*: Ketones act as efficient energy molecules, bridging the gap left by reduced glucose availability and becoming a key energy source for various bodily functions.
- *Adaptation to a Ketogenic State*: Over time, the body adapts to this new metabolic state, efficiently utilizing fats and ketones for sustained energy, marking the achievement of nutritional ketosis.

Understanding this metabolic shift provides a foundation for embracing the benefits of ketosis, including improved fat utilization, steady energy levels, and potential health advantages associated with this alternative metabolic state.

b. Identifying Keto-Friendly Foods

A practical list of keto-friendly foods is provided, outlining items suitable for building meals with the right macronutrient ratios. Clear examples of healthy fats, low-carb vegetables, and protein sources are presented to assist readers in crafting balanced and satisfying meals.

1. Healthy Fats:

- *Avocado*: A nutrient-dense fruit rich in healthy fats, particularly monounsaturated fats.
- *Olive Oil:* An excellent source of monounsaturated fats with a distinct flavor for salad dressings and cooking.
- *Coconut Oil*: Provides medium-chain triglycerides (MCTs), a type of fat easily converted into ketones.
- *Butter/Ghee*: High in saturated fats and suitable for cooking or adding flavor to dishes.
- *Nuts and Seeds* (Almonds, Chia Seeds, Flaxseeds): Packed with healthy fats, fiber, and essential nutrients.

2. Low-Carb Vegetables:

- *Leafy Greens* (Spinach, Kale, Swiss Chard): Low in carbs and high in vitamins, minerals, and antioxidants.

- *Cruciferous Vegetables* (Broccoli, Cauliflower, Brussels Sprouts): Versatile options rich in fiber and nutrients.
- *Zucchini*: A low-carb vegetable that can be spiralized into noodles or added to various dishes.
- *Bell Peppers*: Colorful and flavorful, offering moderate carbs and essential nutrients.
- *Asparagus*: Low in carbs and rich in folate, vitamin K, and antioxidants.

3. Protein Sources:

- *Eggs*: A complete protein source with essential amino acids.
- *Chicken* (Skin-on, Thighs, Breast): Versatile and rich in protein, suitable for various keto recipes.
- *Beef* (Ground, Steak): Provides essential nutrients like iron and zinc.
- *Fish* (Salmon, Tuna, Cod): Rich in omega-3 fatty acids and protein.
- *Tofu and Tempeh*: Plant-based protein sources for those following a vegetarian keto diet.

4. Dairy and Dairy Alternatives:

- *Cheese* (Cheddar, Mozzarella, Cream Cheese): Low-carb and high-fat options for flavor and texture.
- *Heavy Cream:* A keto-friendly addition to coffee or used in sauces and recipes.
- *Greek Yogurt* (Full-Fat): Higher in fat and lower in carbs compared to regular yogurt.
- *Almond Milk/Coconut Milk* (Unsweetened): Low-carb alternatives to regular milk.

5. Condiments and Flavor Enhancers:

- *Olive Tapenade*: Adds flavor and healthy fats to dishes.
- *Mayonnaise* (Avocado Oil or Olive Oil-Based): A rich source of healthy fats.
- *Mustard*: A low-calorie, low-carb condiment to enhance taste.
- *Herbs and Spices:* Flavorful additions with minimal carbs for seasoning.

Crafting meals with a combination of these keto-friendly foods ensures a wellrounded, satisfying, and nutritionally balanced approach to the ketogenic diet. It allows for a diverse and enjoyable culinary experience while adhering to the principles of macronutrient ratios conducive to ketosis.

2. Consulting Healthcare Professionals: Prioritizing Your WellBeing

a.   Importance of Healthcare Consultation

Emphasizing the significance of consulting with a healthcare professional before embarking on a significant dietary change is crucial. Readers are encouraged to discuss their health history, potential contraindications, and individual health goals with a qualified healthcare provider. This step ensures a safe and personalized approach to adopting a keto lifestyle.

b.   Monitoring Health Markers

Guidance on monitoring essential health markers, such as blood glucose levels, cholesterol, and other relevant metrics, is provided. This proactive approach ensures that individuals can track changes, and healthcare professionals can make informed recommendations based on personalized health data.

1. Blood Glucose Levels:

Why Monitor:

- *Objective*: To assess how effectively the body is managing blood sugar.
- *Ketosis Connection:* Fluctuations in blood glucose can impact ketone production.

Monitoring Tips:

- *Regular Testing*: Use a blood glucose monitor to measure levels at different times of the day.
- *Fasting Levels*: Measure fasting blood glucose in the morning before consuming food.
- *Post-Meal Monitoring*: Check levels after meals to observe the body's response to different foods.

Optimal Range:

- *Fasting*: Typically, fasting blood glucose levels below 100 mg/dL are considered normal.
- *Post-Meal:* Aim for levels below 140 mg/dL two hours after eating.

2. Cholesterol Levels:

Why Monitor:

- *Understanding Lipid Profile*: Assess the impact of dietary changes on cholesterol levels. - *Individual Response:* Responses to a keto diet can vary; monitoring helps tailor dietary choices.

Monitoring Tips:

- *Comprehensive Lipid Panel*: Measure total cholesterol, LDL (low-density lipoprotein), HDL (high-density lipoprotein), and triglycerides.
- *Regular Testing*: Periodic testing allows for tracking trends over time.

Optimal Range:

- *LDL and HDL*: The ratio of LDL to HDL is often considered more important than absolute values.
- *Triglycerides*: Aiming for lower levels is generally beneficial.

3. Ketone Levels:

Why Monitor:

- *Confirmation of Ketosis*: Ketone levels indicate the degree of fat burning for energy. - *Individual Variability*: Response to a keto diet can differ; monitoring provides personalized insights.

Monitoring Tips:

    - *Ketone Strips or Meter*: Use urine strips or a blood ketone meter for measurements.
    - *Consistency Matters*: Test at the same time each day for more accurate comparisons.

Optimal Range:

    - *Nutritional Ketosis*: Blood ketone levels between 0.5 to 3.0 mmol/L generally indicate a state of nutritional ketosis.

4. Electrolyte Balance:

Why Monitor:

    - *Common Imbalances*: Sodium, potassium, and magnesium imbalances can occur during keto adaptation.
    - *Preventing Keto Flu:* Monitoring helps address electrolyte deficiencies that may cause symptoms like fatigue or muscle cramps.

Monitoring Tips:

    - *Dietary Sources*: Consume foods rich in electrolytes, such as leafy greens, avocados, and nuts.
    - *Supplementation*: Consider supplements if needed, especially during the initial stages of a keto diet.

Optimal Range:

    - *Individual Needs*: Optimal ranges vary, but maintaining balance is key.

5. General Health Metrics:

Why Monitor:

    - *Comprehensive Well-Being*: Beyond keto-specific markers, monitor general health metrics.
    - *Adaptation Evaluation*: Observe energy levels, mood, and overall vitality.

Monitoring Tips:

    - *Regular Check-ups*: Schedule routine health check-ups with a healthcare professional. - *Symptom Awareness*: Be mindful of changes in energy, mood, digestion, and sleep.

Optimal Range:

    - *Subjective Evaluation*: Look for improvements in overall well-being and the resolution of any pre-existing health concerns.

Regularly monitoring these health markers, in conjunction with consulting a healthcare professional, provides a holistic approach to managing and optimizing health while following a ketogenic diet. Individual responses can vary, so personalized attention to these metrics contributes to a well-informed and sustainable keto journey.

3. Setting Realistic Goals and Expectations: The Key to LongTerm Success

a. Establishing Achievable Objectives

Setting realistic goals is pivotal for sustaining motivation and achieving long-term success. Readers are guided through the process of establishing achievable objectives that align with their individual health aspirations. The focus is on gradual, sustainable progress rather than rapid, short-term changes.

Guide to Setting Achievable Objectives on a Ketogenic Journey:

1. Clarify Your Goals:

- Clearly define your health goals with the ketogenic diet, considering aspects like weight management, improved energy, or blood sugar control.

2. Break Down Goals:

- Divide your long-term vision into smaller, manageable milestones for gradual progress.

3. SMART Goal Setting:

- Ensure your goals are Specific, Measurable, Achievable, Relevant, and TimeBound.

4. Gradual Implementation:

- Introduce changes at a comfortable pace, focusing on developing sustainable habits.

5. Listen to Your Body:

- Pay attention to how your body responds to dietary changes and make adjustments accordingly.

6. Seek Support:

- Consult healthcare professionals and connect with a supportive community for guidance and encouragement.

7. Celebrate Achievements:

- Acknowledge and celebrate your progress, regardless of size, to stay motivated.

8. Long-Term Mindset:

- Shift your perspective from quick fixes to cultivating a sustainable lifestyle with lasting habits.

This concise guide emphasizes a mindful and gradual approach to achieving health goals on a ketogenic journey.

b. Understanding the Adaptation Period

A detailed explanation of the adaptation period—commonly known as the "keto flu"—is provided. Readers are prepared for potential short-term challenges as the body adjusts to the new dietary paradigm. Strategies for mitigating discomfort during this period are outlined, fostering a smoother transition into the keto lifestyle.

Navigating the Adaptation Period on a Keto Journey: Overcoming the "Keto Flu"

Embarking on a ketogenic lifestyle introduces a transitional phase known as the "keto flu," a common experience as the body adjusts to a new dietary paradigm. This section offers a detailed exploration of the adaptation period, equipping readers with insights into potential short-term challenges and providing strategies to ease discomfort for a smoother transition into the keto lifestyle.

Understanding the Keto Flu:

Physiological Shifts: The keto flu occurs as the body undergoes significant metabolic changes. The reduction of carbohydrates prompts a shift from relying on glucose to burning fats for energy, leading to adjustments in fluid balance and electrolyte levels.

Common Symptoms: Readers are informed about potential symptoms, including fatigue, headaches, irritability, and muscle cramps. These are often attributed to dehydration, electrolyte imbalances, and the body's adaptation to using ketones for fuel.

Mitigating Discomfort: Strategies for a Smoother Transition:

Hydration Emphasis:

-       Importance of Water Intake: Readers are encouraged to stay well-hydrated to counteract fluid shifts during the adaptation phase.
-       Electrolyte-Rich Beverages: Introducing beverages rich in electrolytes, such as broth or electrolyte supplements, supports optimal hydration.

Electrolyte Management:

-       Sodium, Potassium, and Magnesium: A focus on increasing intake of these electrolytes helps address imbalances, minimizing symptoms like muscle cramps. - Dietary Sources: Guidance on incorporating electrolyte-rich foods, like leafy greens and avocados, into daily meals.

Gradual Adjustment Approach:

- Slow Carbohydrate Reduction: Suggesting a gradual reduction in carbohydrate intake rather than an abrupt shift can ease the body into ketosis, potentially minimizing the severity of keto flu symptoms.

Adequate Fat Intake:

- Balancing Macros: Emphasizing the importance of consuming enough healthy fats to provide sustained energy during the initial stages of ketosis.

Patience and Self-Care:

- Understanding Variability: Recognizing that individual experiences with the keto flu can vary allows readers to approach the adaptation period with patience. - Rest and Sleep: Stressing the significance of ample rest and quality sleep to support the body's recovery and adaptation.

Consultation with Healthcare Professionals:

- Individual Health Considerations: Encouraging readers to consult with healthcare professionals, particularly if pre-existing health conditions are present or if symptoms persist.

Conclusion: Transitioning with Confidence:

Empowering readers with knowledge about the keto flu and practical strategies for alleviating discomfort ensures they approach the adaptation period with confidence. By navigating this phase mindfully, individuals can optimize their chances of a smoother transition into the enriching and transformative keto lifestyle.

c. Navigating Social and Practical Challenges

Recognizing that lifestyle changes can impact social dynamics and daily routines, practical tips are offered for navigating social gatherings, dining out, and managing practical challenges that may arise. This section aims to equip readers with strategies for maintaining their commitment to keto in various real-life scenarios.

Navigating Social and Practical Challenges on the Keto Journey: Adapting to Real-Life Scenarios

Recognizing that lifestyle changes can impact social dynamics and daily routines, this section provides practical tips for readers on navigating social gatherings, dining out, and managing practical challenges that may arise. The aim is to equip readers with strategies for maintaining their commitment to keto in various real-life scenarios.

Adapting to Social Gatherings:

Communication is Key:

- Encourage open communication with friends and family about your dietary choices.
- Share your commitment to keto and discuss potential meal options beforehand.

Bring Keto-Friendly Dishes:

- Contribute dishes that align with your dietary preferences to ensure there are suitable options available.
- Showcase the delicious and diverse aspects of a ketogenic diet.

Focus on Shared Experiences:

- Emphasize activities and connections beyond food to shift the focus from meals. - Engage in social aspects of gatherings, reinforcing that the event is about more than just what's on the plate.

Dining Out with Confidence:

Review Menus in Advance:

- Research restaurant menus beforehand to identify keto-friendly options. - This allows for informed choices and minimizes potential challenges when ordering.

Customize Your Order:

- Don't hesitate to request modifications to dishes to align with keto principles. - Most establishments are accommodating to dietary preferences.

Choose Wisely, Enjoy Mindfully:

- Opt for dishes rich in healthy fats, proteins, and low-carb vegetables.
- Practice mindful eating to savor the experience without compromising keto goals.

Managing Practical Challenges:

Grocery Shopping Strategies:

- Plan and create a keto-friendly grocery list in advance.
- Stick to the perimeter of the store where fresh produce, meats, and dairy are typically located.

Meal Prep for Success:

- Invest time in weekly meal prep to have keto-friendly options readily available. - This minimizes the temptation to stray from the diet during busy periods.

Stay Hydrated:

- Carry water or other keto-friendly beverages to stay hydrated throughout the day. - Hydration contributes to overall well-being and can aid in managing hunger.

Conclusion: Sustaining Keto Commitment in Real-Life Scenarios:

Empowering readers with practical tips for real-life scenarios ensures they can maintain their commitment to keto amid social gatherings, dining out, and daily challenges. By integrating these strategies, individuals can navigate diverse situations with confidence, making the ketogenic lifestyle an adaptable and sustainable choice.

4. Building a Sustainable Foundation for Keto Success

a. Sustainable Meal Planning on the Keto Journey: A Practical Approach for

Feasibility and Enjoyment

This section offers practical advice on meal planning, providing readers with tips for batch cooking, preparing keto-friendly recipes, and incorporating variety into daily meals. The aim is to assist readers in developing a sustainable approach to meal preparation, ensuring that keto remains feasible and enjoyable in the long run.

Strategies for Effective Meal Planning:

Batch Cooking Benefits:

Batch cooking proves to be a valuable ally on your ketogenic journey, offering the dual benefits of time efficiency and a reliable reservoir of delectable keto-friendly options. This culinary strategy allows for optimized time in the kitchen, reducing the daily cooking grind. By designating specific days for batch cooking, you transform the often stressful routine of meal preparation into a focused and efficient session, minimizing daily kitchen tasks. The advantages extend to consistent access to ketofriendly meals, eliminating the temptation to stray from dietary goals during busy moments. Portion control becomes inherent in the process, as batch cooking allows for pre-portioning meals to align with macronutrient targets. Emphasizing the versatility of batch cooking encourages experimentation with diverse keto recipes, ensuring a week filled with both nutritional and flavorful options. By integrating batch cooking into a routine, readers can effortlessly navigate their keto lifestyle, enjoying the convenience of well-prepared meals throughout the week.

Meal Prepping with Keto in Mind:

Central to a successful ketogenic journey is the strategic planning of meals around keto-friendly ingredients. This emphasis ensures that each meal aligns seamlessly with the principles of the ketogenic diet, promoting a low-carb, high-fat approach. By prioritizing keto-friendly ingredients, individuals can craft meals that not only satisfy their taste buds but also contribute to the attainment of their macronutrient goals. This involves a thoughtful selection of nutrient-dense foods, incorporating a balance of healthy fats, lean proteins, and low-carbohydrate vegetables. This intentional approach to meal creation not only supports nutritional objectives but also enhances the overall effectiveness and sustainability of the ketogenic lifestyle. Through a mindful consideration of ingredients, individuals can cultivate a varied and balanced menu, making each meal a nourishing step toward their health and wellness goals.

Diverse and Nutrient-Rich Recipes:

Encouraging a diverse culinary experience within the realm of ketogenic living involves exploring an array of keto-friendly recipes. By embracing variety, individuals can elevate their meals, making the ketogenic diet a flavorful and enjoyable journey. This entails a creative exploration of recipes that showcase the versatility of ketoapproved ingredients, ensuring a rich and satisfying menu. Furthermore, it underscores the importance of incorporating nutrient-dense foods into the mix. This deliberate focus on nutrient density not only aligns with the principles of the ketogenic diet but also plays a crucial role in promoting overall health. By combining a spectrum of flavors and prioritizing nutrient-rich ingredients, individuals can cultivate a sustainable and wholesome approach to their ketogenic lifestyle, fostering both culinary enjoyment and holistic well-being.

Tips for Practical Implementation:

Weekly Meal Plans:

Facilitating a well-organized and purposeful ketogenic journey involves guiding readers in the creation of weekly meal plans. This strategic approach ensures not only a streamlined and efficient meal preparation process but also helps individuals stay on track with their dietary goals. The emphasis here is on crafting balanced and nutritionally sound meal plans. By suggesting the incorporation of a diverse mix of protein sources, healthy fats, and low-carb vegetables, individuals can enjoy a wellrounded and satisfying array of meals. This variety not only adds richness to the culinary experience but also contributes to balanced nutrition, aligning with the core principles of the ketogenic lifestyle. Through the thoughtful curation of weekly meal plans, individuals can navigate their dietary choices with intention, making each meal a deliberate step toward sustained well-being.

Smart Grocery Shopping:

Streamlining the keto-conscious grocery shopping experience is a key aspect of a successful ketogenic journey. Offering practical tips for efficiency in this endeavor, readers are encouraged to adopt a mindful approach to their grocery lists. Emphasizing the importance of sticking to the perimeters of the store, where fresh produce, meats, and dairy are typically located, ensures a focus on whole and unprocessed foods integral to the ketogenic diet. This strategic shopping advice not only promotes efficiency but also cultivates a conscious selection of nutrient-dense, keto-friendly ingredients. By incorporating these tips into their grocery routine, individuals can confidently navigate the aisles, making intentional choices that align with their dietary preferences and contribute to a successful and sustainable ketogenic lifestyle.

Flexible Approach:

Recognizing the dynamic nature of daily life, the importance of flexibility in meal planning for a ketogenic lifestyle takes center stage. This emphasis extends beyond rigid structures, acknowledging the need to accommodate changing schedules and evolving preferences. By stressing the significance of adaptability, readers are guided to approach meal planning with a fluid mindset. This involves being open to adjustments without compromising the core principles of the ketogenic diet. Providing guidance on how to adapt plans ensures that individuals can navigate unexpected changes while staying true to their keto journey. This flexibility not only fosters a more sustainable approach but also empowers individuals to seamlessly integrate the ketogenic lifestyle into the ever-shifting rhythms of their lives.

Incorporating Variety for Enjoyable Meals:

Exploring Cuisine Diversity:

Inviting a sense of culinary adventure into the ketogenic lifestyle, readers are encouraged to explore a rich variety of cuisines, infusing excitement into their meals. This encouragement to diversify goes beyond the constraints of a traditional approach, emphasizing that different culinary styles can harmoniously align with keto guidelines. By embracing a multitude of flavors and ingredients, individuals can craft a vibrant and interesting menu that transcends the perceived limitations of a specific diet. This exploration not only adds a delightful element to daily meals but also showcases the adaptability of keto principles across a spectrum of global cuisines. Through this culinary exploration, individuals can discover the joy of a diverse and keto-friendly palette, transforming their dietary journey into a captivating and sustainable experience.

Creative Recipe Adaptations:

Igniting a spark of creativity within the realm of keto living, readers are encouraged to infuse innovation into their culinary journey by adapting favorite recipes to align with keto principles. This inspiration lies in the art of transforming beloved dishes into keto-friendly renditions, showcasing the adaptability and versatility of ketoapproved ingredients. The suggestion here is to reimagine traditional recipes, demonstrating that familiar flavors and comfort foods can seamlessly fit within the framework of a ketogenic diet. This creative adaptation not only breathes new life into cherished meals but also underscores the richness and flexibility inherent in the diverse range of keto ingredients. Through this exploration, individuals can savor the joy of reinventing the familiar, turning everyday favorites into keto delights that align with both taste preferences and dietary goals.

Celebrating Food Enjoyment:

At the heart of the ketogenic lifestyle is a celebration of flavors, and readers are encouraged to relish the joy and satisfaction that keto-approved foods can bring to their palates. This reinforcement emphasizes that keto is not just a dietary approach but a flavorful and enjoyable journey. The encouragement extends to savoring the richness and diversity inherent in keto-approved ingredients. By reveling in the vibrant tastes and textures of wholesome fats, proteins, and low-carb vegetables, individuals can cultivate a deeper appreciation for the delicious array of foods that align with the principles of the ketogenic diet. This mindful savoring of flavors underscores the pleasure and satisfaction that can be derived from every ketofriendly bite, making the dietary experience not only health-conscious but also a source of culinary delight.

Conclusion: Long-Term Feasibility and Enjoyment

Empowering readers with practical meal planning advice ensures they can seamlessly integrate keto into their lifestyle. By emphasizing batch cooking, diverse recipes, and flexible approaches, individuals can maintain a sustainable relationship with the ketogenic diet, making it not just a temporary choice but a long-term, enjoyable commitment.

b. Grocery Shopping Guidance

Navigating the grocery store through a keto lens involves a thoughtful and informed approach, empowering individuals to make choices aligned with their ketogenic journey. Begin by exploring the perimeters of the store, where fresh produce, meats, and dairy are usually located. Focus on nutrient-dense, whole foods that are the backbone of a keto diet. When venturing into the aisles, carefully read food labels to identify hidden sugars and high-carb ingredients. A comprehensive list of ketofriendly foods becomes your guide, including an array of fresh vegetables, quality meats, poultry, fish, eggs, dairy, nuts, and healthy fats. Emphasize whole, unprocessed options, and consider adding low-carb substitutes for traditional items. By adopting this strategic approach to grocery shopping, individuals can seamlessly integrate keto principles into their dietary choices, making the shopping experience not just a routine but a mindful step towards a nourishing and satisfying keto lifestyle.

CHAPTER 4: UNDERSTANDING MACRONUTRIENTS

The journey into the ketogenic lifestyle begins with a profound comprehension of macronutrients—carbohydrates, fats, and proteins—each playing a pivotal role in achieving the goals of women over 60 embarking on a keto diet.

Section 1: Roles of Macronutrients in the Keto Diet

In this section, we unravel the distinctive roles of carbohydrates, fats, and proteins within the ketogenic framework. Understanding how each macronutrient contributes to energy metabolism and overall well-being forms the foundation for a successful keto journey.

Carbohydrates:

Embarking on the ketogenic journey entails a transformative shift from the conventional reliance on carbohydrates as the primary energy source to embracing a low-carb lifestyle. The significance of this transition lies in the initiation and sustenance of ketosis, a metabolic state where the body efficiently burns fats for fuel instead of carbohydrates.

By restricting carbohydrate intake, individuals trigger a cascade of metabolic changes that lead to the production of ketones, serving as an alternative energy source derived from fats. This shift not only promotes efficient fat burning but also offers a range of potential health benefits, including improved weight management, increased mental clarity, and enhanced energy levels.

Central to the success of this transition is the emphasis on the quality of carbohydrates when they are included. Rather than indiscriminately slashing all carbs, the focus is on choosing nutrient-dense, whole-food sources that contribute valuable vitamins, minerals, and fiber. Opting for complex carbohydrates found in vegetables, nuts, and seeds ensures a steady release of energy without causing drastic spikes in blood sugar levels.

Highlighting the importance of nutrient-dense carbs reinforces the idea that not all carbohydrates are created equal. This nuanced approach enables individuals to make informed choices, selecting carbohydrates that align with their nutritional goals and contribute to overall well-being. In essence, this exploration underscores the transformative power of embracing a low-carb lifestyle, where mindful carbohydrate choices play a pivotal role in the success and sustainability of the ketogenic journey.

Fats:

Delving into the heart of the ketogenic diet, fats emerge as the unsung heroes, serving as the primary energy source during the state of ketosis. Contrary to some misconceptions surrounding fat consumption, the ketogenic approach champions the integration of healthy fats as a cornerstone for sustained energy and overall health.

In ketosis, the body undergoes a metabolic shift, prioritizing the breakdown of fats into ketones for energy rather than relying on glucose from carbohydrates. This not only facilitates efficient fat burning but also provides a stable and enduring source of energy, promoting endurance and mental clarity.

Dispelling myths about fat consumption is crucial in this narrative. The emphasis here is on distinguishing between healthy and unhealthy fats. Rather than fearing fats as a dietary villain, the ketogenic lifestyle encourages the incorporation of nutrientdense and heart-healthy fats. Avocados, nuts, and olive oil stand out as exemplary sources, rich in monounsaturated and polyunsaturated fats, which contribute to cardiovascular health and overall well-being.

By embracing these healthy fats, individuals on the ketogenic journey not only support their energy needs but also nourish their bodies with essential nutrients. This nuanced approach to fat consumption not only aligns with the core principles of the ketogenic diet but also dismantles misconceptions, empowering individuals to make informed and health-conscious choices for a sustainable and fulfilling ketogenic lifestyle.

Proteins:

In the journey through the keto landscape for women over 60, proteins assume a crucial role. Beyond the aesthetic aspects, they become the architects of muscle preservation, contributing to metabolic health and overall functional well-being. Proteins extend their influence, supporting vital bodily functions, from enzymes to hormones, fortifying the foundations of health as we age. Navigating the optimal protein intake becomes nuanced, tailored to the unique needs of women in their 60s, balancing muscle preservation with the intricacies of effective ketosis. Guiding the selection of high-quality protein sources—lean meats, fish, eggs, and plant-based options—empowers readers to make proteins a cornerstone of their keto experience, enriching the journey with nutrient-dense choices that contribute not just to daily vitality but to sustained well-being.

Section 2: Tailoring Macronutrient Ratios for Women Over 60

Recognizing the unique health considerations of women over 60, we offer tailored guidelines for macronutrient ratios in the keto journey. In this demographic, a balanced approach takes precedence, acknowledging the significance of nuanced recommendations to support metabolic health and overall well-being. The emphasis is on a personalized strategy, considering factors such as age-related metabolic changes, health milestones, and specific concerns prevalent in this life stage. Tailoring macronutrient ratios ensures a fine-tuned balance, promoting not only effective ketosis but also addressing the distinctive health needs of women over 60. This approach fosters a sense of empowerment, guiding individuals in optimizing their nutritional intake for a keto journey that aligns seamlessly with their health aspirations and the intricacies of this specific demographic.

Section 3: Practical Guidance with Food Examples

Facilitating a seamless integration into daily life, let's explore a diverse array of food examples for each macronutrient category, tailored for the nutritional needs of women over 60 on a keto journey.

Low-carb Vegetables:

Think of vibrant leafy greens like spinach and kale, cruciferous vegetables such as broccoli and cauliflower, and colorful bell peppers. These nutrient-dense options not only bring a spectrum of vitamins and minerals but also contribute minimal carbohydrates, allowing for a satisfying and health-conscious inclusion in daily meals.

Lean Proteins:

For lean protein sources, consider skinless poultry like chicken or turkey, fatty fish such as salmon and trout, and plant-based options like tofu or tempeh. These choices provide essential amino acids while maintaining a balance in protein intake, crucial for muscle preservation and overall bodily functions.

Wholesome Fats:

When it comes to wholesome fats, avocados, nuts, and olive oil take center stage.

Avocados offer creamy richness and heart-healthy monounsaturated fats, while nuts provide a satisfying crunch along with beneficial nutrients. Olive oil, a staple in the Mediterranean diet, not only enhances flavors but also contributes to overall wellbeing.

These examples empower women over 60 to make informed and enjoyable food

choices, aligning seamlessly with their keto goals. By incorporating this diverse array of nutrient-dense foods, individuals can craft a flavorful and nourishing diet that supports their health aspirations and enhances their overall well-being on the keto path.

In conclusion, Chapter 4 acts as a beacon of understanding, guiding women over 60 through the intricacies of macronutrients on their keto journey. By demystifying the roles of carbohydrates, fats, and proteins, and providing tailored guidelines and practical food examples, this chapter equips readers with the knowledge and confidence needed to embark on a personalized and successful ketogenic lifestyle.

CHAPTER5: KETO-FRIENDLY FOODS FOR WOMEN OVER 60

In this chapter, we embark on a comprehensive exploration of keto-friendly foods curated to suit the unique needs of women over 60. Recognizing the importance of nutrient-dense, whole foods, we delve into the rich tapestry of options that align seamlessly with a keto lifestyle. Additionally, we offer valuable tips for grocery shopping and meal planning, ensuring a practical and enjoyable approach to integrating these foods into daily life.

Comprehensive List of Keto-Friendly Foods:

1. *Low-Carb Vegetables*: Spinach, kale, broccoli, cauliflower, zucchini, and bell peppers.
2. *Lean Proteins*: Chicken, turkey, salmon, trout, tofu, and tempeh.
3. *Healthy Fats*: Avocados, nuts (almonds, walnuts), olive oil, and coconut oil.
4. *Dairy*: Greek yogurt, cheese, and butter (preferably from grass-fed sources).
5. *Eggs*: A versatile and protein-rich option.
6. *Berries*: Limited quantities of strawberries, blueberries, and raspberries for a touch of sweetness.
7. *Herbs and Spices*: Flavor enhancers that add zest without compromising ketosis.

Importance of Nutrient-Dense, Whole Foods:

Understanding that nutrient density is paramount, we emphasize the significance of whole foods. These choices not only contribute essential vitamins and minerals but also support overall health. Nutrient-dense options provide a robust foundation for women over 60, addressing specific health considerations and promoting vitality through the keto journey.

Tips for Grocery Shopping and Meal Planning:

1. *Plan Ahead*: Outline meals for the week and create a shopping list to streamline the grocery shopping process.
2. *Focus on Fresh Produce*: Prioritize fresh, seasonal vegetables and fruits to enhance variety and nutritional intake.
3. *Read Labels*: When choosing packaged items, scrutinize labels for hidden sugars and unnecessary additives.
4. *Experiment with Recipes*: Keep meal planning exciting by trying new keto recipes that incorporate diverse flavors and ingredients.

This chapter serves as a practical guide, offering not just a list of keto-friendly foods but insights into the importance of nutrient-dense choices. By providing tips for grocery shopping and meal planning, we aim to empower women over 60 with the tools to make informed, enjoyable, and health-conscious decisions on their keto journey.

CHAPTER 6: NAVIGATING THE KETO PATH-MISTAKESAND SOLUTIONSFOR BEGINNERS

Embarking on a keto journey can be transformative, yet it's not without its pitfalls, especially for beginners. In this chapter, we unravel common mistakes made by those new to the keto diet and provide practical strategies to sidestep these challenges, ensuring a smoother and more successful entry into the world of ketosis.

Common Mistakes:

1. Overlooking Hidden Carbs: Many beginners unknowingly consume hidden carbohydrates, often found in sauces, dressings, or processed foods. These hidden carbs can impede progress into ketosis.

Avoiding the oversight of hidden carbs demands a vigilant approach to food choices. Developing the habit of meticulously reading nutrition labels becomes a cornerstone in this endeavor, enabling individuals to identify and understand the carbohydrate content of various products. It involves a shift in mindset, prompting a heightened awareness of ingredients in sauces, dressings, or processed foods where hidden carbs often lurk. Cultivating a routine of mindful eating, where attention is paid to both ingredients and nutritional information, acts as a safeguard against unintentional carb consumption. This proactive and informed approach empowers individuals to make conscious choices, reducing the likelihood of overlooking hidden carbs and supporting a more successful adherence to the ketogenic lifestyle.

2. Inadequate Hydration: Failing to prioritize hydration can lead to electrolyte imbalances, commonly known as the "keto flu," resulting in fatigue, headaches, and muscle cramps.

Preventing inadequate hydration on the keto journey necessitates a proactive commitment to regular and mindful fluid intake. It goes beyond a mere suggestion; it's a fundamental practice for overall well-being. Begin by cultivating the habit of consistently drinking water throughout the day, aiming for a sufficient daily intake. Infusing variety by incorporating herbal teas or incorporating flavored water can make hydration more appealing. Additionally, paying attention to signs of thirst and incorporating hydrating foods, such as water-rich vegetables, into meals contributes to overall fluid balance. By making hydration a conscious and integral part of daily routines, individuals can mitigate the risk of inadequate fluid intake, ensuring a smooth and comfortable experience as they navigate the ketogenic lifestyle.

3. Ignoring Nutrient Diversity: Some beginners may focus solely on fats and neglect the importance of a well-rounded, nutrient-dense diet, which can lead to deficiencies.

Steering clear of neglecting nutrient diversity requires a deliberate shift towards appreciating the holistic aspects of the keto lifestyle. It involves more than a casual recommendation; it's a commitment to understanding the nutritional value of diverse foods. Begin by broadening the spectrum of food choices, incorporating an array of colorful vegetables, various protein sources, and healthy fats into meals. Cultivate an adventurous approach to cooking and experimenting with different recipes to ensure a variety of nutrients are present. Regularly reassessing and adjusting the composition of meals helps avoid monotony and ensures a comprehensive range of essential vitamins and minerals. By embracing nutrient diversity as a core principle, individuals elevate their keto experience, promoting overall health and well-being through a rich and varied nutritional intake.

4. *Imbalanced Macronutrient Ratios*: Striking the right balance between fats, proteins, and carbs is crucial. Beginners may inadvertently skew their macronutrient ratios, hindering the body's transition into ketosis.

Guarding against imbalanced macronutrient ratios necessitates a conscientious approach to meal planning and nutritional awareness. It's not just advice; it's a strategic effort to maintain the delicate balance required for successful ketosis. Begin by setting clear macronutrient goals based on individual needs and adjusting them as necessary. Actively choose a variety of whole foods that contribute to the right balance of fats, proteins, and carbohydrates. Regularly tracking and reassessing macronutrient intake ensures alignment with the desired ratios. By incorporating this intentional approach into daily dietary choices, individuals can sidestep the pitfalls of imbalanced macronutrients, fostering a more effective and sustainable experience with the ketogenic lifestyle.

5. *Lack of Planning*: Failure to plan meals and snacks can lead to impulsive, non-keto food choices, undermining progress and causing frustration.

Steering clear of the pitfalls associated with a lack of planning requires a strategic approach to meal preparation and decision-making. This isn't merely a suggestion; it's a proactive stance to ensure a smooth journey on the keto lifestyle. Start by dedicating time to plan meals in advance, considering nutritional requirements and personal preferences. Create a weekly menu, outline a shopping list, and prep ingredients to minimize impulsive decisions. Cultivate the habit of having ketofriendly snacks readily available, reducing the likelihood of reaching for noncompliant options when hunger strikes. By integrating planning into the routine, individuals fortify their commitment to the ketogenic lifestyle, setting the stage for success through intentional and informed choices.

Strategies and Solutions:

1.   *Read Labels:* Navigating the intricacies of a keto lifestyle begins with empowering beginners to unravel the mysteries of hidden carbs and decipher nutrition labels. Understanding the subtle presence of carbohydrates concealed in sauces, dressings, or processed foods is key to making informed choices. By instilling this foundational knowledge, individuals gain a sharper awareness of their dietary selections, enabling them to navigate the complex landscape of the keto journey with confidence. Reading nutrition labels becomes an art form, equipping beginners with the skills needed to discern between keto-friendly options and those that may derail their path to ketosis. This newfound proficiency lays the groundwork for a successful and sustainable embrace of the ketogenic lifestyle.

2.   *Prioritize Hydration*: Ensuring that you stay well-hydrated is absolutely crucial, especially as you embark on your journey into the keto lifestyle. Let's emphasize the significance of maintaining a consistent intake of fluids throughout the day. Hydration is not only about water but also involves paying attention to your electrolyte balance, a key factor in avoiding the potential challenges often associated with starting

keto, known as the "keto flu." To support this, consider incorporating nourishing options like broth or electrolyte supplements into your routine. This emphasis on hydration lays a strong foundation for your overall well-being, making your transition into the ketogenic lifestyle smoother and more comfortable.

3. *Encourage Nutrient-Rich Foods*: Emphasizing the diversity of keto-friendly, nutrientdense foods is a foundational principle for ensuring a broad spectrum of essential vitamins and minerals in your diet. This emphasis goes beyond a mere suggestion; it's a strategy designed to guarantee a comprehensive and balanced nutritional intake. By actively incorporating a variety of nutrient-dense options into your meals, you're not just enhancing taste and texture but also providing your body with a wealth of vital nutrients. This focus on diversity stands as a practical and enjoyable approach to nourishing your body, unlocking the full benefits of the ketogenic lifestyle for your overall health and well-being.

4. *Guidance on Tracking Macros*: Navigating the intricacies of a keto lifestyle involves a crucial element – tracking macronutrients. For beginners, this practice is more than just a suggestion; it's a practical tool to maintain the optimal balance for successful ketosis. By actively monitoring the intake of fats, proteins, and carbohydrates, individuals gain a nuanced understanding of their dietary composition. Practical tips, such as using dedicated apps or journals, empower beginners to make informed choices, ensuring their macronutrient ratios align with the requirements of the ketogenic journey. This proactive approach not only fosters a sense of control but also sets the stage for a more effective and rewarding experience with the keto lifestyle.

5. *Meal Planning:* Stressing the significance of meal planning is paramount in the realm of the keto lifestyle, offering a structured approach to sidestep impulsive decisions. This isn't just a suggestion; it's a practical strategy to ensure steadfast adherence to the principles of the ketogenic journey. By proactively planning meals, individuals create a roadmap for their dietary choices, minimizing the risk of succumbing to non-keto options in moments of spontaneity. This intentional approach not only fosters discipline but also makes the keto lifestyle more sustainable and enjoyable. Through meal planning, individuals empower themselves to navigate daily choices with purpose, reinforcing their commitment to the principles of ketosis and cultivating a positive and successful experience with the ketogenic lifestyle.

This chapter serves as a valuable roadmap for beginners, equipping them with the knowledge to sidestep common pitfalls on their keto journey. By addressing these mistakes and providing effective solutions, we aim to empower beginners with the tools for a successful and sustainable experience with the ketogenic lifestyle.

CHAPTER 7: MEAL PLANNING AND RECIPES

In this chapter, we embark on a flavorful exploration of meal planning and recipes tailored for the dynamic needs of women over 60 in their keto journey.

Sample Meal Plans:

Discover thoughtfully crafted meal plans covering breakfast, lunch, dinner, and snacks. These plans serve as practical guides, providing a diverse range of options that align with the nutritional requirements of this demographic. Each meal plan is designed to make keto not just a diet but a delightful culinary experience.

Delightful Culinary Adventures: Sample Meal Plans

Embark on a culinary journey designed specifically for the vibrant women over 60 embracing the keto lifestyle. Our thoughtfully crafted meal plans offer not just nourishment but a delightful fusion of flavors and nutrition.

Breakfast:

Start your day with a burst of energy and satisfaction. Our breakfast options combine the richness of healthy fats with the freshness of nutrient-dense ingredients, ensuring you kickstart your morning in the best possible way.

Breakfast Bliss: Energize Your Mornings

Elevate your mornings with our specially curated breakfast options, designed to infuse your day with a burst of energy and satisfaction. We believe that the first meal of the day should not only fuel your body but also be a delightful experience.

Our breakfast selections artfully combine the richness of healthy fats with the freshness of nutrient-dense ingredients. Picture starting your day with creamy avocado and smoked salmon, a perfect harmony of omega-3s and satisfying fats. Alternatively, relish the simplicity of a fluffy omelet generously filled with vibrant vegetables, providing essential nutrients to kickstart your morning.

These breakfast choices go beyond the ordinary; they are crafted to ensure you not only meet your nutritional needs but also relish the flavors that define the essence of the keto lifestyle. Whether you prefer savory or sweet, these breakfast options transform your mornings into a delightful ritual, setting the tone for a day filled with vitality and joy. Because, for us, breakfast is more than a meal – it's a celebration of the delicious possibilities that keto living brings to your table.

1. Avocado and Smoked Salmon Delight:

- Ingredients:
- Ripe avocado

- Smoked salmon slices
- Fresh dill - Lemon wedge
- Preparation:
- Slice the avocado and arrange it on a plate.
- Drape smoked salmon over the avocado slices.
- Garnish with fresh dill and a squeeze of lemon for a zesty touch.

2. Vegetable-Packed Omelet:

- Ingredients:
- Eggs
- Bell peppers (various colors), diced
- Spinach leaves
- Feta cheese (optional)
- Olive oil
- Preparation:
- Whisk eggs and pour them into a heated pan with olive oil.
- Add diced bell peppers and spinach to the eggs.
- Once cooked, fold the omelet and sprinkle with feta cheese if desired.

3. Chia Seed Pudding Parfait:

- Ingredients:
- Chia seeds
- Unsweetened almond milk
- Berries (strawberries, blueberries, raspberries)
- Slivered almonds - Preparation:
- Mix chia seeds with almond milk and let it sit in the refrigerator overnight.
- In the morning, layer the chia pudding with fresh berries and top with slivered almonds.

4. Keto-friendly Smoothie Bowl: - Ingredients:
- Unsweetened almond milk
- Mixed berries (blueberries, raspberries)
- Spinach leaves - Chia seeds - Almond butter - Preparation:
- Blend almond milk, berries, spinach, and a spoon of almond butter until smooth.
- Pour into a bowl and sprinkle chia seeds for added texture.

5. Greek Yogurt Parfait: - Ingredients:
- Full-fat Greek yogurt
- Walnuts or almonds
- Dark chocolate shavings (85% cocoa or higher)
- Vanilla extract - Preparation:
- Layer Greek yogurt with nuts and a dash of vanilla extract. - Top with dark chocolate shavings for a decadent touch.

6. Egg and Bacon Breakfast Muffins:
- Ingredients: - Eggs

- Bacon strips
- Spinach leaves - Cherry tomatoes, halved - Preparation:
- Line muffin cups with bacon strips.
- Crack an egg into each cup, add spinach and a tomato half. - Bake until eggs are set for a savory breakfast delight.

Dive into these morning creations, where each bite not only aligns with keto goodness but also brings a symphony of flavors to your breakfast table. These options provide the perfect balance of healthy fats and nutrient density, ensuring your mornings are not just energetic but also a joyous celebration of delicious keto living.

These breakfast ideas not only introduce variety to your mornings but also ensure you enjoy the richness of healthy fats and the goodness of nutrient-dense ingredients. Embrace these recipes as a delightful way to begin your day on a keto high note.

Lunch:

Savor satisfying and easy-to-prepare lunches that cater to both taste and nutritional needs. These meals provide a perfect balance of macronutrients, keeping you fueled and focused throughout the day.

Lunchtime Harmony: Fulfilling Your Keto Cravings

Midday nourishment becomes an art form with our selection of lunches that seamlessly blend satisfaction with nutritional excellence. These meals are not just about fueling your body; they are a harmonious fusion of taste and nutrients, providing a perfect balance of macronutrients to keep you energized and focused throughout the day.

1. Salmon and Avocado Salad:

- Ingredients:
- Grilled salmon fillet
- Mixed salad greens
- Avocado slices
- Cherry tomatoes
- Olive oil and lemon dressing - Preparation:
- Arrange grilled salmon on a bed of mixed greens.
- Add avocado slices and cherry tomatoes.
- Drizzle with olive oil and a squeeze of fresh lemon for a refreshing touch.
2. Chicken and Broccoli Stir-Fry: - Ingredients:
- Sliced chicken breast
- Broccoli florets
- Bell peppers (sliced)
- Coconut aminos or soy sauce
- Sesame oil
- Preparation:

- Stir-fry chicken in sesame oil until cooked.
- Add broccoli and bell peppers, cooking until vegetables are tender. - Season with coconut aminos for a flavorful stir-fry.
  3. Zucchini Noodles with Pesto and Cherry Tomatoes:
- Ingredients:
- Zucchini noodles (zoodles)
- Homemade or store-bought pesto
- Cherry tomatoes, halved - Parmesan cheese (optional) - Preparation:
- Sauté zucchini noodles until just tender.
- Toss with pesto sauce and top with cherry tomatoes.
- Sprinkle with Parmesan if desired for a light and flavorful lunch.

4. Egg Salad Lettuce Wraps:

- Ingredients:
- Hard-boiled eggs, chopped
- Avocado
- Dijon mustard
- Lettuce leaves for wrapping - Preparation:
- Mash avocado and mix with chopped eggs and Dijon mustard.
- Spoon the mixture onto lettuce leaves for a refreshing and satisfying wrap.

5. Shrimp and Vegetable Skewers:

- Ingredients:
- Shrimp, peeled and deveined
- Cherry tomatoes
- Zucchini, sliced
- Olive oil and lemon marinade - Preparation:
- Thread shrimp, cherry tomatoes, and zucchini onto skewers.
- Grill or bake, brushing with olive oil and lemon marinade for a flavorful and protein-packed lunch.

6. Cauliflower Fried Rice with Chicken:

- Ingredients:
- Cauliflower rice

-

-

Cooked chicken breast, diced

- Mixed vegetables (peas, carrots, and corn)
- Coconut aminos or soy sauce

Preparation:

- Sauté cauliflower rice, diced chicken, and mixed vegetables.
- Season with coconut aminos or soy sauce for a low-carb twist on fried rice.

These lunch options not only satiate your taste buds but also provide a well-rounded mix of macronutrients, ensuring you stay fueled and focused as you navigate the demands of your day. Lunchtime becomes a delightful pause in your routine, where you not only nourish your body but also revel in the joy of flavors on your keto journey.

Dinner:

Indulge in dinners that transform ordinary meals into extraordinary experiences. These keto-friendly recipes are not just about restriction; they're about reveling in the joy of culinary exploration while supporting your health goals.

Evening Elegance: Transformative Keto Dinners

Dinnertime takes on a new dimension with our collection of keto-friendly recipes that elevate ordinary meals into extraordinary culinary experiences. These dinner options go beyond mere restriction; they invite you to revel in the joy of culinary exploration while steadfastly supporting your health goals.

1. Grilled Steak with Garlic Butter: - Ingredients:
- Ribeye or sirloin steak
- Garlic cloves, minced
- Butter
- Fresh parsley, chopped - Preparation:
- Grill the steak to your preferred doneness.
- In a pan, melt butter and sauté minced garlic until fragrant.
- Pour the garlic butter over the grilled steak and sprinkle with fresh parsley.
2. Cauliflower Crust Pizza:
- Ingredients:
- Cauliflower crust (store-bought or homemade)
- Sugar-free tomato sauce
- Mozzarella cheese
- Your favorite pizza toppings (pepperoni, olives, mushrooms) - Preparation:
- Spread tomato sauce on the cauliflower crust.
- Add mozzarella cheese and your desired toppings. - Bake until the cheese is melted and bubbly.

3. Salmon and Asparagus Foil Packets:

- Ingredients:
- Salmon fillets
- Asparagus spears
- Lemon slices - Dill, fresh or dried - Preparation:
- Place salmon and asparagus on a foil sheet.
- Season with lemon slices and dill.
- Seal the foil packet and bake for a flavorful and fuss-free dinner.
4. Chicken Alfredo Zucchini Noodles: - Ingredients:
- Zucchini noodles (zoodles)
- Cooked chicken breast, sliced
- Alfredo sauce (keto-friendly)
- Parmesan cheese - Preparation:
- Sauté zucchini noodles until tender.
- Combine with sliced chicken and keto-friendly Alfredo sauce.
- Garnish with Parmesan cheese for a comforting and low-carb pasta alternative.
5. Stuffed Bell Peppers with Ground Turkey:
- Ingredients:
- Bell peppers, halved
- Ground turkey
- Cauliflower rice - Tomato sauce (sugar-free) - Preparation:
- Brown ground turkey and mix with cauliflower rice.
- Fill bell pepper halves with the turkey mixture.

Bake with sugar-free tomato sauce for a wholesome stuffed pepper dish.

6. Vegetarian Eggplant Lasagna:

Ingredients:

- Eggplant, thinly sliced
- Ricotta cheese
- Spinach leaves
- Marinara sauce (sugar-free) - Preparation:
- Layer eggplant slices with ricotta and spinach.
- Top with sugar-free marinara sauce.
- Bake until bubbly for a delectable vegetarian lasagna.

These dinner recipes are a testament to the pleasure of keto dining, where each bite is an invitation to savor the richness of flavors while staying true to your health journey. Whether you're grilling a steak, crafting a cauliflower crust pizza, or enjoying a simple yet elegant foil packet, these dinner options turn ordinary evenings into extraordinary moments of keto delight.

-

-

Snacks:

Enjoy guilt-free snacking with our curated selection of keto-friendly snacks. From savory to sweet, each snack is a testament to the delicious possibilities within the ketogenic realm.

Snacking Delights: Guilt-Free Keto Bites

Satisfy your cravings without derailing your keto journey with our handpicked selection of guilt-free, keto-friendly snacks. From savory to sweet, each bite is a testament to the delicious possibilities that the ketogenic realm has to offer.

1. Cheese and Pepperoni Bites: - Ingredients:
   - Mozzarella cheese cubes
   - Pepperoni slices - Cherry tomatoes (optional) - Preparation:
   - Skewer mozzarella cheese cubes with pepperoni slices.
   - Add cherry tomatoes for a burst of freshness.
2. Avocado Chocolate Mousse:
   - Ingredients:
   - Ripe avocados
   - Unsweetened cocoa powder
   - Erythritol or stevia
   - Vanilla extract - Preparation:
   - Blend avocados with cocoa powder, sweetener, and vanilla extract. - Chill for a velvety chocolate mousse.

3. Spiced Almonds:

   - Ingredients: - Almonds
   - Olive oil
   - Paprika, cayenne pepper, and salt - Preparation:
   - Toss almonds with olive oil and a blend of spices.
   - Roast until golden brown for a crunchy, spiced snack.

4. Cucumber and Cream Cheese Rolls:

   - Ingredients:
   - Cucumber, thinly sliced
   - Cream cheese - Smoked salmon (optional) - Preparation:
   - Spread cream cheese on cucumber slices.
   - Roll up and add a slice of smoked salmon for an elegant keto snack.

5. Berries and Whipped Cream:

   - Ingredients:

- Mixed berries (strawberries, blueberries, raspberries)
- Heavy whipping cream
- Vanilla extract - Preparation:
- Whip heavy cream with vanilla extract until soft peaks form.
- Serve with a mix of fresh berries for a delightful, low-carb treat.

6. Bacon-Wrapped Jalapeño Poppers:

- Ingredients:

Jalapeño peppers, halved and seeded

- Cream cheese
- Bacon strips Preparation:
- Fill jalapeño halves with cream cheese.
- Wrap with bacon strips and bake until crispy for a spicy and savory snack.

These keto-friendly snacks not only keep you on track but also elevate your snacking experience. Whether you're reaching for cheese and pepperoni bites, indulging in avocado chocolate mousse, or savoring spiced almonds, these snacks are a delicious celebration of the variety and tastefulness that keto snacking has to offer.

These sample meal plans transcend the conventional notion of dieting. They are meticulously designed to ensure you not only meet your nutritional requirements but relish every bite, making the keto lifestyle a delightful and sustainable part of your daily routine. It's not just about what you eat; it's about the joy and satisfaction each meal brings, making your journey into keto a flavorful and enjoyable adventure.

Portion Control:

Balancing Act: The Importance of Portion Control in Keto Living

Embark on a journey of understanding the pivotal role of portion control in maintaining a harmonious and balanced keto lifestyle. This section unravels the significance of managing serving sizes, providing practical tips that empower individuals to relish their meals while safeguarding their macronutrient goals.

In the world of keto, where precision matters, portion control becomes a guiding principle. It's not about restriction but about finding the equilibrium that keeps you on track with your nutritional objectives. Through insightful tips and practical advice, this section aims to demystify portion control, ensuring that every bite is a step toward both enjoyment and adherence to your keto journey.

Mastering Portion Control in Your Keto Journey

In the realm of keto living, mastering the art of portion control is a cornerstone for success. It's not just about how much you eat, but about finding the right balance to support your macronutrient goals while savoring every bite.

Practical Tips for Portion Control:

1.   Listen to Your Body:

Tune in to your body's hunger and fullness cues. Eating mindfully allows you to recognize when you've had enough, preventing overindulgence.

2.   Use Smaller Plates and Bowls:

Trick your mind into satisfaction by opting for smaller dishes. This visual illusion can make reasonable portions appear more satisfying.

3.   Divide Your Plate:

Mentally divide your plate into sections for proteins, fats, and vegetables. This simple strategy helps ensure a balanced distribution of essential nutrients.

4.   Pre-Portion Snacks:

When it comes to snacks, pre-portioning is key. Package snacks in individual servings to avoid mindless munching and maintain control over your carb and calorie intake.

5.   Mind the Condiments:

Be mindful of condiments and dressings, as they can add up quickly. Use measuring spoons to control portions and avoid unknowingly exceeding your daily carb limits.

6.   Stay Hydrated:

Sometimes, the body may signal hunger when it's actually thirsty. Stay hydrated to distinguish between hunger and thirst, aiding in more accurate portion control.

Remember, portion control in keto isn't about deprivation; it's a strategy for sustainable and enjoyable eating. These practical tips empower you to navigate your keto journey with confidence, ensuring that each portion contributes to your overall well-being.

50 Keto Recipes and 28-Day Meal Plan:

Embark on a culinary journey with a wealth of options – 50 keto recipes spanning breakfast, lunch, and dinner. These recipes not only add variety to your daily meals but also cater to the unique tastes and

-

-

nutritional needs of women over 60. Additionally, discover a comprehensive 28-day meal plan, offering a structured approach to guide individuals through a month of delicious and keto-compliant eating.

50 Keto Recipes:

1. Baked Parmesan Crusted Salmon:

   - Ingredients:
   - Salmon fillets
   - Parmesan cheese, grated
   - Almond flour
   - Garlic powder
   - Dried oregano - Salt and pepper
   - Instructions:
   1. Preheat the oven to 400°F (200°C).
   2. In a bowl, mix grated Parmesan, almond flour, garlic powder, dried oregano, salt, and pepper.
   3. Coat each salmon fillet with the Parmesan mixture.
   4. Place the coated fillets on a baking sheet.
   5. Bake for 12-15 minutes or until the salmon is cooked through and the crust is golden brown.

2. Mushroom and Spinach Stuffed Chicken Breasts:

   - Ingredients:
   - Chicken breasts
   - Mushrooms, chopped
   - Spinach, chopped
   - Cream cheese
   - Garlic powder - Salt and pepper
   - Instructions:
   1. Preheat the oven to 375°F (190°C).
   2. In a pan, sauté mushrooms and spinach until wilted. Add garlic powder, salt, and pepper.
   3. Butterfly the chicken breasts and spread cream cheese inside.
   4. Spoon the mushroom and spinach mixture onto one side of each chicken breast.
   5. Fold the other side over the filling, securing with toothpicks if needed.
   6. Bake for 25-30 minutes or until the chicken is cooked through.

3. Zucchini Noodle Alfredo:

   - Ingredients:
   - Zucchini noodles (Zoodles)
   - Heavy cream
   - Butter
   - Parmesan cheese, grated
   - Garlic powder - Salt and pepper
   - Instructions:

1. In a pan, melt butter and add heavy cream, garlic powder, salt, and pepper.
2. Stir in grated Parmesan until the sauce is smooth.
3. Add zucchini noodles and toss until coated and heated through.
4. Cauliflower Fried Rice with Shrimp:

- Ingredients:
- Cauliflower rice
- Shrimp, peeled and deveined
- Mixed vegetables (peas, carrots, etc.)
- Soy sauce (low-sodium)
- Garlic, minced
- Sesame oil
- Eggs, beaten
- Green onions, chopped (for garnish)
- Instructions:

1. In a wok or skillet, heat sesame oil and sauté garlic.
2. Add shrimp and cook until pink, then add mixed vegetables.
3. Push the mixture to one side and scramble eggs on the other side.
4. Combine everything, add cauliflower rice, and stir in soy sauce.
5. Cook until the cauliflower rice is tender.
6. Garnish with chopped green onions.

5. Eggplant Lasagna Rolls:

- Ingredients:
- Eggplant, thinly sliced
- Ricotta cheese
- Spinach, chopped
- Marinara sauce (sugar-free)
- Mozzarella cheese, shredded
- Parmesan cheese, grated
- Instructions:

1. Preheat the oven to 375°F (190°C).
2. Grill or bake eggplant slices until tender.
3. In a bowl, mix ricotta and chopped spinach.
4. Spread the ricotta mixture onto each eggplant slice and roll them up.
5. Place the rolls in a baking dish, top with marinara sauce and cheeses.
6. Bake for 20-25 minutes or until the cheese is bubbly.

6. Avocado and Bacon Egg Cups:

- Ingredients:
- Avocados, halved and pitted
- Eggs
- Bacon strips - Salt and pepper

- Instructions:
  1. Preheat the oven to 375°F (190°C).
  2. Scoop out a small portion of each avocado half to create a well.
  3. Place the avocado halves in a baking dish to prevent tipping.
  4. Crack an egg into each avocado well.
  5. Wrap each avocado with a bacon strip, securing it around the circumference.
  6. Bake for 15-20 minutes or until the egg is cooked to your liking.
  7. Grilled Portobello Mushrooms with Pesto:
- Ingredients:
- Portobello mushrooms
- Olive oil
- Garlic, minced
- Fresh basil, chopped
- Pine nuts
- Parmesan cheese, grated
- Instructions:
  1. Preheat the grill or oven to medium-high heat.
  2. In a bowl, mix olive oil, minced garlic, chopped basil, pine nuts, and grated Parmesan to make pesto.
  3. Brush the portobello mushrooms with the pesto mixture.
  4. Grill or bake the mushrooms until tender, about 8-10 minutes.

8. Keto Taco Bowls:

- Ingredients:
- Ground beef
- Taco seasoning (low-carb)
- Lettuce, shredded
- Tomatoes, diced
- Cheese, shredded
- Avocado, sliced
- Instructions:
  1. In a skillet, brown ground beef and season with low-carb taco seasoning according to package instructions.
  2. Assemble taco bowls with shredded lettuce as the base.
  3. Top with seasoned ground beef, diced tomatoes, shredded cheese, and sliced avocado.

9. Lemon Garlic Butter Shrimp:

- Ingredients:
- Shrimp, peeled and deveined
- Butter
- Garlic, minced
- Lemon juice

- Fresh parsley, chopped
- Salt and pepper
- Instructions:
1. In a pan, melt butter and sauté minced garlic until fragrant.
2. Add shrimp to the pan and cook until pink.
3. Squeeze fresh lemon juice over the shrimp, season with salt, pepper, and garnish with chopped parsley.

10. Cabbage and Sausage Skillet:

- Ingredients:
- Cabbage, sliced
- Sausage links, sliced
- Onion, thinly sliced
- Garlic, minced
- Paprika - Salt and pepper
- Instructions:
  1. In a large skillet, sauté sliced sausage until browned.
  2. Add minced garlic and sliced onions, cooking until softened.
  3. Incorporate sliced cabbage, season with paprika, salt, and pepper.
  4. Cook until the cabbage is tender, stirring occasionally.

11. Garlic Butter Steak Bites: - *Ingredients*:
- Sirloin steak, cut into bite-sized pieces
- Butter
- Garlic, minced
- Fresh rosemary, chopped
- Salt and pepper
- Instructions:
  1. In a skillet, melt butter and sauté minced garlic until fragrant.
  2. Add steak bites, cooking until browned on all sides.
  3. Sprinkle with chopped rosemary, season with salt and pepper.

12. Spinach and Feta Stuffed Chicken Thighs:
- Ingredients:
- Chicken thighs, boneless and skinless
- Spinach, chopped
- Feta cheese, crumbled
- Garlic powder
- Lemon zest - Salt and pepper
- Instructions:
  1. Preheat the oven to 375°F (190°C).
  2. In a bowl, mix chopped spinach, crumbled feta, garlic powder, and lemon zest.
  3. Stuff each chicken thigh with the spinach and feta mixture.
  4. Bake for 25-30 minutes or until the chicken is cooked through.

13. Shrimp and Asparagus Stir-Fry:

- Ingredients:
- Shrimp, peeled and deveined
- Asparagus, trimmed and cut into pieces
- Soy sauce (low-sodium)
- Ginger, minced
- Sesame oil - Red pepper flakes
- Instructions:
1. In a wok or skillet, heat sesame oil and sauté minced ginger.
2. Add shrimp and cook until pink, then add asparagus pieces.
3. Stir in low-sodium soy sauce and red pepper flakes, cooking until asparagus is tender.

14. Caprese Salad Skewers:

- Ingredients:
- Cherry tomatoes
- Mozzarella balls
- Fresh basil leaves
- Balsamic glaze
- Olive oil - Salt and pepper
- Instructions:
  1. Thread cherry tomatoes, mozzarella balls, and fresh basil leaves onto skewers.
  2. Drizzle with olive oil and balsamic glaze.
  3. Sprinkle with salt and pepper before serving.

15. Keto Meatball Zoodle Bowl:

- Ingredients:
- Zucchini noodles (Zoodles)
- Ground beef
- Almond flour
- Parmesan cheese, grated
- Italian seasoning - Marinara sauce (sugar-free) - *Instructions*:
1. In a bowl, mix ground beef, almond flour, grated Parmesan, and Italian seasoning.
2. Form meatballs and cook until browned.
3. Toss zucchini noodles in marinara sauce and top with meatballs.

16. Bacon-Wrapped Brussels Sprouts:

- Ingredients:
- Brussels sprouts, trimmed
- Bacon strips
- Olive oil

- Garlic powder - Salt and pepper
- Instructions:
1. Preheat the oven to 400°F (200°C).
2. Wrap each Brussels sprout with a bacon strip and secure with a toothpick.
3. Place on a baking sheet, drizzle with olive oil, and season with garlic powder, salt, and pepper.
4. Bake for 20-25 minutes or until the bacon is crispy.

17. Greek Chicken Souvlaki Skewers:

- Ingredients:
- Chicken breasts, cut into cubes
- Greek yogurt
- Lemon juice
- Garlic, minced
- Oregano
- Cucumber, diced (for Tzatziki)
- Instructions:
1. In a bowl, marinate chicken cubes in Greek yogurt, lemon juice, minced garlic, and oregano.
2. Thread marinated chicken onto skewers and grill until cooked.
3. Serve with diced cucumber and homemade Tzatziki sauce.

18. Keto Egg Roll in a Bowl:

- Ingredients:
- Ground pork or turkey
- Coleslaw mix (cabbage and carrots)
- Ginger, minced
- Garlic, minced
- Soy sauce (low-sodium)
- Sesame oil
- Green onions, chopped
- Instructions:
1. In a skillet, brown ground pork or turkey.
2. Add coleslaw mix, minced ginger, and garlic, cooking until vegetables are tender.
3. Stir in low-sodium soy sauce, sesame oil, and chopped green onions.

19. Coconut Curry Chicken:

- Ingredients:
- Chicken thighs, boneless and skinless
- Coconut milk
- Curry powder
- Turmeric
- Garlic, minced

- Ginger, grated - Fresh cilantro, chopped - *Instructions*:
  1. In a pan, sauté minced garlic and grated ginger.
  2. Add chicken thighs and brown on both sides.
  3. Pour in coconut milk, curry powder, and turmeric.

20. Avocado and Bacon Stuffed Chicken Breast:

   - Ingredients:
   - Chicken breasts
   - Avocado, mashed
   - Bacon strips
   - Garlic powder
   - Paprika - Salt and pepper
   - Instructions:
   1. Preheat the oven to 375°F (190°C).
   2. Cut a pocket into each chicken breast.
   3. Fill each pocket with mashed avocado.
   4. Wrap each chicken breast with bacon strips and season with garlic powder, paprika, salt, and pepper.
   5. Bake until chicken is cooked through and bacon is crispy.

21. Eggplant Lasagna:

   - Ingredients:
   - Eggplant, thinly sliced
   - Ground beef or Italian sausage
   - Marinara sauce (sugar-free)
   - Ricotta cheese
   - Mozzarella cheese, shredded
   - Parmesan cheese, grated
   - Italian seasoning - *Instructions*:
   1. Preheat the oven to 375°F (190°C).
   2. In a skillet, brown ground beef or Italian sausage.
   3. Layer sliced eggplant, meat, marinara sauce, ricotta, mozzarella, and Parmesan in a baking dish.
   4. Repeat layers and sprinkle with Italian seasoning.
   5. Bake until bubbly and golden.

22. Pesto Zoodle Bowl with Grilled Chicken:

   - Ingredients:
   - Zucchini noodles (Zoodles)
   - Grilled chicken breast, sliced
   - Cherry tomatoes, halved
   - Pesto sauce

- Pine nuts - Fresh basil leaves - *Instructions*:
  1. Sauté zucchini noodles until tender.
  2. Toss with grilled chicken, cherry tomatoes, and pesto sauce.
  3. Top with pine nuts and fresh basil leaves.

23. Teriyaki Salmon:

- Ingredients:
- Salmon fillets
- Soy sauce (low-sodium)
- Mirin
- Garlic, minced
- Ginger, grated
- Sesame seeds - Green onions, sliced
- Instructions:
  1. In a bowl, mix low-sodium soy sauce, mirin, minced garlic, and grated ginger.
  2. Marinate salmon fillets in the mixture.
  3. Grill or bake until salmon is flaky.
  4. Sprinkle with sesame seeds and sliced green onions.

24. Buffalo Cauliflower Bites: - *Ingredients*:
- Cauliflower florets
- Almond flour
- Garlic powder
- Onion powder
- Buffalo sauce - Ghee or butter
- Instructions:
1. Preheat the oven to 450°F (230°C).
2. In a bowl, coat cauliflower florets with almond flour, garlic powder, and onion powder.
3. Bake until cauliflower is golden.
4. Toss in a mixture of buffalo sauce and melted ghee.

25. Zesty Lemon Herb Chicken Thighs:
- Ingredients:
- Chicken thighs, bone-in and skin-on
- Lemon zest
- Fresh herbs (rosemary, thyme, or oregano), chopped
- Olive oil
- Garlic, minced - Salt and pepper
- Instructions:
1. Preheat the oven to 375°F (190°C).
2. In a bowl, mix lemon zest, chopped herbs, olive oil, minced garlic, salt, and pepper.
3. Coat chicken thighs with the mixture and bake until golden and cooked through.

26. Taco Stuffed Bell Peppers:

- Ingredients:
- Bell peppers, halved
- Ground turkey or beef
- Taco seasoning
- Cherry tomatoes, diced
- Shredded cheese - Fresh cilantro, chopped - *Instructions*:
1. Preheat the oven to 375°F (190°C).
2. Brown ground turkey or beef with taco seasoning.
3. Fill halved bell peppers with the meat mixture, top with diced tomatoes, shredded cheese, and chopped cilantro.
4. Bake until peppers are tender.

27. Creamy Garlic Parmesan Mushrooms:

- Ingredients:
- Mushrooms, cleaned and halved
- Heavy cream
- Parmesan cheese, grated
- Garlic, minced
- Butter
- Fresh parsley, chopped - *Instructions*:
   1. In a skillet, sauté mushrooms in butter until golden.
   2. Add minced garlic and cook until fragrant.
   3. Pour in heavy cream and grated Parmesan, stirring until creamy.
   4. Garnish with chopped fresh parsley.

28. Mediterranean Chicken Skewers:

- Ingredients:
- Chicken breast, cut into cubes
- Cherry tomatoes
- Red onion, sliced
- Kalamata olives
- Feta cheese, crumbled
- Olive oil
- Lemon juice
- Oregano
- Instructions:
   1. Marinate chicken cubes in olive oil, lemon juice, and oregano.
   2. Thread chicken, cherry tomatoes, red onion, and Kalamata olives onto skewers.
   3. Grill until chicken is cooked, then sprinkle with crumbled feta.

29. Keto Tuna Salad Lettuce Wraps:

- Ingredients:
- Canned tuna, drained
- Mayonnaise
- Dijon mustard
- Celery, diced
- Pickles, chopped
- Lettuce leaves - *Instructions*:
1. In a bowl, mix canned tuna, mayonnaise, Dijon mustard, diced celery, and chopped pickles.
2. Spoon the tuna salad into lettuce leaves to create wraps.

30. Sausage and Vegetable Skillet:

    - Ingredients:
    - Sausages, sliced
    - Bell peppers, sliced
    - Zucchini, sliced
    - Onion, sliced
    - Italian seasoning
    - Olive oil
    - Instructions:
1. In a skillet, brown sliced sausages in olive oil.
2. Add sliced bell peppers, zucchini, and onion, sautéing until vegetables are tender.
3. Season with Italian seasoning and serve.

31. Grilled Shrimp and Asparagus Skewers:

    - Ingredients:
    - Shrimp, peeled and deveined
    - Asparagus spears
    - Olive oil
    - Lemon juice
    - Garlic, minced - Salt and pepper
    - Instructions:
1. Marinate shrimp and asparagus in a mixture of olive oil, lemon juice, minced garlic, salt, and pepper.
2. Thread onto skewers and grill until shrimp are pink and asparagus is tender.

32. Cabbage and Ground Beef Stir-Fry:

    - Ingredients:
    - Ground beef
    - Cabbage, shredded
    - Soy sauce (low-sodium)
    - Sesame oil

- Ginger, grated
- Garlic, minced
- Green onions, sliced
- Instructions:
  1. In a skillet, brown ground beef.
  2. Add shredded cabbage, soy sauce, sesame oil, grated ginger, and minced garlic.
  3. Stir-fry until cabbage is tender, then garnish with sliced green onions.

33. Caprese Salad with Balsamic Glaze:

- Ingredients:
- Cherry tomatoes, halved
- Fresh mozzarella, sliced
- Fresh basil leaves
- Balsamic glaze
- Olive oil - Salt and pepper
- Instructions:
  1. Arrange cherry tomatoes, mozzarella slices, and fresh basil on a plate.
  2. Drizzle with olive oil and balsamic glaze.
  3. Season with salt and pepper.

34. Lemon Garlic Butter Shrimp:

- Ingredients:
- Shrimp, peeled and deveined
- Butter
- Garlic, minced
- Lemon juice
- Fresh parsley, chopped
- Salt and pepper
- Instructions:
  1. In a skillet, melt butter and sauté minced garlic.
  2. Add shrimp and cook until pink.
  3. Drizzle with lemon juice, sprinkle with chopped fresh parsley, and season with salt and pepper.

35. Egg Roll in a Bowl:

- Ingredients:
- Ground pork or turkey
- Coleslaw mix
- Soy sauce (low-sodium)
- Ginger, grated
- Garlic, minced
- Sesame oil - Green onions, sliced

- Instructions:
  1. Brown ground pork or turkey in a skillet.
  2. Add coleslaw mix, soy sauce, grated ginger, minced garlic, and sesame oil.
  3. Stir-fry until the coleslaw is tender, then garnish with sliced green onions.

36. Stuffed Bell Peppers with Ground Turkey:

- Ingredients:
- Bell peppers, halved
- Ground turkey
- Cauliflower rice
- Tomato sauce (sugar-free)
- Italian seasoning
- Mozzarella cheese, shredded - *Instructions*:
1. Preheat the oven to 375°F (190°C).
2. Brown ground turkey, then mix with cauliflower rice, tomato sauce, and Italian seasoning.
3. Fill halved bell peppers, top with shredded mozzarella, and bake until peppers are tender.

37. Spinach and Feta Stuffed Chicken Breast:

- Ingredients:
- Chicken breasts
- Spinach, wilted and chopped
- Feta cheese, crumbled
- Garlic powder
- Olive oil - Salt and pepper
- Instructions:
1. Preheat the oven to 375°F (190°C).
2. Make a pocket in each chicken breast and stuff with wilted spinach and crumbled feta.
3. Season with garlic powder, olive oil, salt, and pepper, then bake until chicken is cooked through.

38. Shrimp and Broccoli Alfredo:

- Ingredients:
- Shrimp, peeled and deveined
- Broccoli florets
- Heavy cream
- Parmesan cheese, grated
- Garlic, minced
- Butter
- Instructions:
  1. In a skillet, cook shrimp and broccoli in butter and minced garlic.
  2. Pour in heavy cream and grated Parmesan, stirring until creamy.

39. Greek Salad with Grilled Chicken:

- Ingredients:
- Grilled chicken breast, sliced
- Mixed greens
- Cucumber, sliced
- Cherry tomatoes, halved
- Kalamata olives
- Feta cheese, crumbled
- Red onion, thinly sliced
- Olive oil
- Red wine vinegar
- Oregano
- Instructions:
1. Assemble mixed greens, cucumber, cherry tomatoes, Kalamata olives, feta cheese, and red onion.
2. Top with grilled chicken slices.
3. Drizzle with olive oil, red wine vinegar, and sprinkle with oregano.

40. Zucchini Noodles with Pesto and Cherry Tomatoes:

- Ingredients:
- Zucchini noodles (Zoodles)
- Pesto sauce
- Cherry tomatoes, halved
- Pine nuts
- Parmesan cheese, grated
- Instructions:
  1. Sauté zucchini noodles until tender.
  2. Toss with pesto sauce and cherry tomatoes.
  3. Garnish with pine nuts and grated Parmesan.

41. Avocado and Bacon Egg Cups:

- Ingredients:
- Avocados, halved and pitted
- Eggs
- Bacon strips
- Salt and pepper
- Chives, chopped (optional) - *Instructions*:
1. Preheat the oven to 375°F (190°C).
2. Place avocado halves in a baking dish.
3. Crack an egg into each avocado half, wrap with bacon strips, and bake until eggs are set.
4. Season with salt and pepper, garnish with chopped chives if desired.

42. Cauliflower Mac and Cheese:

- Ingredients:
- Cauliflower florets
- Heavy cream
- Cream cheese
- Cheddar cheese, shredded
- Mustard powder
- Paprika - Salt and pepper
- Instructions:
1. Steam cauliflower until tender.
2. In a saucepan, mix heavy cream, cream cheese, shredded cheddar, mustard powder, paprika, salt, and pepper until smooth.
3. Combine with cauliflower for a keto-friendly mac and cheese.

43. Pecan-Crusted Salmon:

- Ingredients:
- Salmon fillets
- Pecans, finely chopped
- Dijon mustard
- Olive oil
- Lemon zest
- Salt and pepper
- Instructions:
1. Preheat the oven to 400°F (200°C).
2. Mix finely chopped pecans, Dijon mustard, olive oil, lemon zest, salt, and pepper.
3. Coat salmon fillets with the pecan mixture and bake until salmon is cooked through.

44. Buffalo Chicken Lettuce Wraps:

- Ingredients:
- Shredded chicken
- Buffalo sauce
- Lettuce leaves
- Celery, diced
- Blue cheese crumbles - Ranch dressing (optional) - *Instructions*:
1. Mix shredded chicken with buffalo sauce.
2. Spoon the buffalo chicken into lettuce leaves.
3. Top with diced celery, blue cheese crumbles, and a drizzle of ranch dressing if desired.

45. Eggplant Lasagna:

- Ingredients:

- Eggplant, thinly sliced
- Ground beef or turkey
- Low-carb marinara sauce
- Ricotta cheese
- Mozzarella cheese, shredded
- Parmesan cheese, grated
- Italian seasoning - *Instructions*:

1. Preheat the oven to 375°F (190°C).
2. Brown ground beef or turkey, layer with sliced eggplant, marinara sauce, ricotta, and shredded mozzarella.
3. Repeat layers, sprinkle with Parmesan and Italian seasoning, and bake until bubbly.

46. Cilantro Lime Chicken Thighs:

- Ingredients:
- Chicken thighs
- Fresh cilantro, chopped
- Lime juice
- Garlic, minced
- Olive oil - Salt and pepper
- Instructions:

1. Marinate chicken thighs in a mixture of chopped cilantro, lime juice, minced garlic, olive oil, salt, and pepper.
2. Grill or bake until chicken is cooked through.

47. Turkey and Zucchini Skillet:

- Ingredients:
- Ground turkey
- Zucchini, diced
- Onion, diced
- Garlic, minced
- Italian seasoning
- Tomato sauce (sugar-free)
- Olive oil
- Instructions:

1. In a skillet, brown ground turkey in olive oil with diced zucchini, onion, and minced garlic.
2. Season with Italian seasoning, add sugar-free tomato sauce, and simmer until flavors meld.

48. Keto Tuna Salad Lettuce Wraps:

- Ingredients:
- Canned tuna, drained
- Mayonnaise (sugar-free)

- Dill pickles, chopped
- Celery, diced - Lettuce leaves - *Instructions*:
  1. Mix tuna with sugar-free mayonnaise, chopped dill pickles, and diced celery.
  2. Spoon tuna salad into lettuce leaves for refreshing wraps.

49. Zesty Lemon Butter Cauliflower Rice:

- Ingredients:
- Cauliflower rice
- Butter
- Lemon juice
- Lemon zest
- Parsley, chopped
- Salt and pepper
- Instructions:
1. Sauté cauliflower rice in butter until tender.
2. Drizzle with lemon juice, sprinkle with lemon zest, chopped parsley, salt, and pepper.

50. Chocolate Avocado Mousse:

- Ingredients:
- Avocado
- Cocoa powder (unsweetened)
- Heavy cream
- Vanilla extract
- Monk fruit sweetener (or sweetener of choice)
- Instructions:
1. Blend avocado, unsweetened cocoa powder, heavy cream, vanilla extract, and sweetener until smooth.
2. Chill before serving for a rich and creamy chocolate mousse.

These recipes provide a delicious variety for your keto culinary adventure. If you have any specific preferences or adjustments, feel free to make them to your liking!

28 Day Meal Plan

Embark on a transformative 28-day keto journey with our carefully crafted meal plan designed to not just fuel your body but elevate your entire well-being. Meal planning is the cornerstone of a successful keto lifestyle, offering structure, variety, and the assurance that every bite aligns with your health goals. This comprehensive plan introduces you to a delightful array of keto-friendly recipes, emphasizing nutrientdense, whole foods tailored to women over 60. Beyond fostering physical health, meal planning instills discipline and cultivates a positive relationship with food, paving the way for sustained success on your keto adventure. Embrace the joy of culinary exploration as you navigate this thoughtfully curated 28-day meal plan, making keto not just a diet but a sustainable and enjoyable way of life.

Week 1:

Day 1:

- Breakfast: Avocado and Bacon Egg Cups
- Lunch: Turkey and Zucchini Skillet
- Dinner: Pecan-Crusted Salmon - Snack: Keto Tuna Salad Lettuce Wraps

Day 2:

- Breakfast: Cauliflower Mac and Cheese
- Lunch: Chicken Caesar Salad (without croutons)
- Dinner: Eggplant Lasagna
- Snack: Zesty Lemon Butter Cauliflower Rice

Day 3:

- Breakfast: Chocolate Avocado Mousse
- Lunch: Buffalo Chicken Lettuce Wraps
- Dinner: Cilantro Lime Chicken Thighs - Snack: Keto Tuna Salad Lettuce Wraps

Day 4:

- Breakfast: Keto Tuna Salad Lettuce Wraps
- Lunch: Turkey and Zucchini Skillet
- Dinner: Avocado and Bacon Egg Cups
- Snack: Chocolate Avocado Mousse

Day 5:

- Breakfast: Pecan-Crusted Salmon
- Lunch: Eggplant Lasagna
- Dinner: Buffalo Chicken Lettuce Wraps - Snack: Zesty Lemon Butter Cauliflower Rice

Day 6:

- Breakfast: Chocolate Avocado Mousse - Lunch: Cauliflower Mac and Cheese
- Dinner: Cilantro Lime Chicken Thighs - Snack: Keto Tuna Salad Lettuce Wraps

Day 7:

- Breakfast: Avocado and Bacon Egg Cups
- Lunch: Chicken Caesar Salad (without croutons)
- Dinner: Zesty Lemon Butter Cauliflower Rice - Snack: Buffalo Chicken Lettuce Wraps

Week 2:

Day 8:

- Breakfast: Keto Tuna Salad Lettuce Wraps
- Lunch: Zesty Lemon Butter Cauliflower Rice
- Dinner: Buffalo Chicken Lettuce Wraps - Snack: Chocolate Avocado Mousse

Day 9:

- Breakfast: Pecan-Crusted Salmon
- Lunch: Avocado and Bacon Egg Cups
- Dinner: Chicken Caesar Salad (without croutons) - Snack: Keto Tuna Salad Lettuce Wraps

Day 10:

- Breakfast: Chocolate Avocado Mousse
- Lunch: Cilantro Lime Chicken Thighs
- Dinner: Eggplant Lasagna
- Snack: Buffalo Chicken Lettuce Wraps

Day 11:

- Breakfast: Avocado and Bacon Egg Cups
- Lunch: Turkey and Zucchini Skillet
- Dinner: Cauliflower Mac and Cheese - Snack: Zesty Lemon Butter Cauliflower Rice

Day 12:

- Breakfast: Chocolate Avocado Mousse
- Lunch: Keto Tuna Salad Lettuce Wraps
- Dinner: Pecan-Crusted Salmon - Snack: Buffalo Chicken Lettuce Wraps

Day 13:

- Breakfast: Zesty Lemon Butter Cauliflower Rice
- Lunch: Chicken Caesar Salad (without croutons)
- Dinner: Avocado and Bacon Egg Cups - Snack: Keto Tuna Salad Lettuce Wraps

Day 14:

- Breakfast: Cauliflower Mac and Cheese
- Lunch: Buffalo Chicken Lettuce Wraps
- Dinner: Cilantro Lime Chicken Thighs - Snack: Chocolate Avocado Mousse

Week 3:

Day 15:

- Breakfast: Keto Blueberry Chia Seed Pudding
- Lunch: Shrimp and Avocado Salad
- Dinner: Beef and Broccoli Stir-Fry - Snack: Cucumber and Cream Cheese Bites

Day 16:

- Breakfast: Spinach and Feta Omelette
- Lunch: Chicken and Vegetable Skewers
- Dinner: Zucchini Noodles with Pesto and Cherry Tomatoes - Snack: Keto Avocado Chocolate Mousse

Day 17:

- Breakfast: Keto Almond Flour Pancakes
- Lunch: Caprese Salad with Balsamic Glaze
- Dinner: Salmon with Lemon-Dill Sauce - Snack: Pepperoni and Cheese Roll-Ups

Day 18:

- Breakfast: Keto Green Smoothie
- Lunch: Cobb Salad with Avocado
- Dinner: Cabbage Wrapped Ground Beef Enchiladas - Snack: Deviled Eggs with Bacon

Day 19:

- Breakfast: Keto Cheddar and Chive Muffins
- Lunch: Tuna Zoodle Casserole
- Dinner: Grilled Portobello Mushrooms with Garlic Butter - Snack: Keto Chocolate Hazelnut Fat Bombs

Day 20:

- Breakfast: Avocado and Bacon Egg Muffins
- Lunch: Greek Salad with Feta
- Dinner: Keto Chicken Alfredo with Zucchini Noodles - Snack: Smoked Salmon Cucumber Rolls

Day 21:

- Breakfast: Keto Coconut Flour Waffles
- Lunch: Turkey and Avocado Lettuce Wraps
- Dinner: Pork Tenderloin with Rosemary Roasted Radishes - Snack: Keto Mixed Berry Yogurt Parfait

Week 4:

Day 22:

- Breakfast: Keto Pumpkin Spice Chia Pudding
- Lunch: Spinach and Bacon Stuffed Chicken Breast
- Dinner: Zucchini Noodles Aglio e Olio with Shrimp - Snack: Keto Lemon Poppy Seed Fat Bombs

Day 23:

- Breakfast: Keto Berry Protein Smoothie
- Lunch: Egg Salad Lettuce Wraps
- Dinner: Grilled Chicken Thighs with Garlic Butter Asparagus - Snack: Avocado and Bacon Deviled Eggs

Day 24:

- Breakfast: Keto Cinnamon Roll Mug Cake
- Lunch: Avocado and Shrimp Salad
- Dinner: Beef and Vegetable Kebabs - Snack: Chocolate Mint Keto Fat Bombs

Day 25:

- Breakfast: Keto Chocolate Chia Pudding
- Lunch: Caesar Salad with Grilled Salmon
- Dinner: Lemon Herb Baked Cod - Snack: Keto Caprese Skewers

Day 26:

- Breakfast: Keto Sausage and Egg Breakfast Casserole
- Lunch: Turkey and Avocado Roll-Ups
- Dinner: Baked Garlic Parmesan Chicken Wings - Snack: Keto Raspberry Cheesecake Bites

Day 27:

- Breakfast: Keto Almond Butter and Jelly Muffins
- Lunch: Cucumber and Smoked Salmon Salad
- Dinner: Cauliflower Fried Rice with Shrimp - Snack: Pecan Pie Keto Fat Bombs

Day 28:

- Breakfast: Keto Blueberry Pancake Stack
- Lunch: Chicken Caesar Lettuce Wraps
- Dinner: Grilled Lamb Chops with Rosemary Cauliflower Mash
- Snack: Keto Peanut Butter Chocolate Chip Cookies

Maintain variety by incorporating different recipes or repeating your favorites. Feel free to experiment with additional keto-friendly meals and snacks to keep your 28day keto journey exciting and enjoyable! Remember to adjust portion sizes based on your individual needs and consult with a healthcare professional if needed. Enjoy your 28-day keto journey!

CHAPTER8:OVERCOMING CHALLENGES

Navigating the keto journey is a commendable endeavor, yet challenges may arise along the way. In this chapter, we'll confront common hurdles head-on and equip you with practical strategies for overcoming them. Cravings, a frequent companion on any dietary path, are addressed with tailored approaches to keep them at bay. We delve into the social intricacies of dining out and provide strategies for seamlessly integrating keto into various social situations. Additionally, we shed light on potential side effects, ensuring you're well-prepared to mitigate them effectively. By proactively tackling these challenges, you'll not only overcome obstacles but also foster a sustainable and successful keto experience.

Cravings

Cravings, those ever-present companions on any dietary journey, merit a nuanced approach to ensure they're effectively managed. Recognizing that cravings often arise from a combination of psychological, emotional, and physiological factors, implementing tailored strategies becomes key. One effective tactic is to identify and address the root cause of cravings. Are they triggered by stress, emotions, or perhaps certain habits? By understanding these triggers, you can develop personalized coping mechanisms, such as mindful practices, stress reduction techniques, or indulging in satisfying keto-friendly alternatives.

Dining out, a social fabric woven into our lives, demands a strategic yet enjoyable approach when following a keto lifestyle. Consider it an opportunity for culinary exploration rather than a challenge. Embrace restaurant menus with a discerning eye, seeking out options rich in grilled proteins, leafy greens, and nourishing fats. Don't hesitate to communicate your dietary preferences to restaurant staff; many establishments are more than willing to accommodate specific requests, ensuring a satisfying and keto-compliant dining experience.

Social gatherings, often centered around shared meals, might pose unique challenges. However, with a bit of planning, you can seamlessly integrate keto into various social situations. Prioritize satiety by enjoying a satisfying keto meal before attending events, making it easier to resist non-keto temptations. Additionally, consider bringing keto-friendly dishes to share, showcasing the delicious diversity of the ketogenic lifestyle. Open communication with friends and family about your dietary choices fosters understanding and support, turning social occasions into opportunities for shared enjoyment.

Remember, the journey is not only about adhering to a diet but about crafting a lifestyle that aligns with your health goals. By navigating cravings and social intricacies with intention and creativity, you'll find that the keto lifestyle becomes a sustainable and fulfilling part of your social experiences.

Potential Side-Effects

Embarking on the keto journey can bring about certain side effects, and being wellprepared to navigate them is an integral part of a successful experience. One commonly encountered phenomenon is the "keto flu," a set of symptoms that some individuals may experience during the initial stages of adapting to a ketogenic diet. These symptoms, ranging from fatigue and headaches to irritability, are typically transient as your body adjusts to utilizing fat for energy. Ensuring you stay adequately hydrated, maintaining electrolyte balance through sources like broth or supplements, and gradually easing into the keto lifestyle can contribute significantly to alleviating these transitional discomforts.

Another aspect to be mindful of is the potential impact on bowel habits. The substantial shift in dietary composition, particularly the increase in fats and reduction in carbs, can influence digestive patterns. To mitigate this, consider introducing fiber-rich foods gradually, stay well-hydrated, and explore the inclusion of probiotics to support a healthy gut.

Changes in sleep patterns might also be observed during the initial stages of keto adaptation. While some individuals report improvements in sleep quality, others may experience alterations. Establishing a consistent sleep routine, creating a conducive sleep environment, and incorporating relaxation techniques before bedtime can help optimize your sleep experience.

It's crucial to recognize that responses to the keto diet are highly individualized. If you encounter persistent or severe side effects, seeking guidance from a healthcare professional is advisable. Their expertise can provide personalized insights and recommendations tailored to your specific needs, ensuring a smoother and more comfortable journey on the keto lifestyle. By shedding light on potential side effects and adopting proactive mitigation strategies, you're not just embarking on a diet but embracing a transformative and well-informed lifestyle.

CHAPTER9:STAYINGACTIVEANDFIT

In the pursuit of a vibrant and healthful life, staying active is paramount, especially for women over 60. This chapter underscores the profound significance of physical activity in promoting overall well-being and longevity. Engaging in regular exercise not only contributes to physical health but also positively influences mental and emotional wellness.

For women in this age group, it's essential to tailor exercise routines to suit individual needs and capabilities. Suggesting appropriate exercise routines involves incorporating a mix of aerobic exercises, strength training, flexibility exercises, and balance-enhancing activities. These elements collectively contribute to maintaining a well-rounded fitness regimen that supports bone health, muscle strength, and overall physical function.

Understanding the symbiotic relationship between exercise and the keto diet is crucial. Physical activity complements the metabolic benefits of the keto lifestyle, enhancing fat utilization for energy and promoting weight management. As the body becomes more efficient at burning fat, coupled with the muscle-preserving effects of exercise, women over 60 can experience improved body composition and functional fitness.

This chapter serves as a guide to empower women in their 60s to embrace a lifestyle where the synergy between the keto diet and regular exercise becomes a cornerstone of their well-being. It's not just about movement; it's about fostering strength, resilience, and an active enjoyment of life well into the golden years.

Physical Activity

Physical activity holds a profound significance in promoting overall well-being and longevity, extending its impact far beyond just physical health. Engaging in regular exercise becomes a holistic approach to nurturing not only the body but also the mind and emotions.

1.   **Physical Health Benefits:** Regular exercise is a cornerstone of maintaining physical health, contributing to cardiovascular health, optimal weight management, and enhanced muscular and skeletal strength. It plays a pivotal role in preventing and managing various health conditions, including heart disease, diabetes, and osteoporosis. The cardiovascular benefits of exercise, such as improved blood circulation and heart function, are instrumental in supporting overall longevity.

2.   **Mental Well-Being:** Physical activity is a powerful ally for mental health. Exercise stimulates the release of endorphins, often referred to as "feel-good" hormones, which contribute to a sense of happiness and well-being. Additionally, regular exercise has been linked to improved cognitive function, memory, and a reduced risk of neurodegenerative conditions. It provides a natural way to manage stress and anxiety, fostering mental resilience.

3.   **Emotional Wellness:** The emotional benefits of exercise extend to managing mood and reducing the risk of depression. Physical activity offers a positive outlet for emotional energy, promoting a sense of accomplishment and self-esteem. Engaging in exercise also provides an opportunity for social

interaction, whether through group classes, walking clubs, or other communal activities, further contributing to emotional well-being.

4.   **Quality of Life:** Beyond preventing illness, physical activity enhances the overall quality of life. It improves functional abilities, making daily tasks easier and more enjoyable. For individuals in their 60s and beyond, maintaining mobility, flexibility, and balance through exercise is particularly crucial, supporting an active and independent lifestyle.

In essence, regular exercise is a holistic prescription for a longer, healthier, and more fulfilling life. It not only contributes to physical health but also acts as a potent elixir for mental and emotional well-being. The profound impact of physical activity extends far beyond the gym or the jogging path—it becomes a cornerstone for embracing life with vitality and resilience.

Tailoring Exercise Routines

Tailoring exercise routines to suit individual needs and capabilities is essential for several reasons, recognizing the unique characteristics and considerations that individuals bring to their fitness journey:

1.   **Individualized Fitness Levels**: Everyone starts from a different fitness baseline. Tailoring exercise routines allows individuals to begin at a level that is challenging yet achievable for them. This approach ensures that the exercise is neither too strenuous nor too easy, promoting gradual progress.

2.   **Health Considerations:** Individuals may have varying health conditions, previous injuries, or specific health goals. Customizing exercise routines allows for considerations of these factors. For example, someone with joint concerns might benefit from low-impact exercises, while strength training could be particularly crucial for individuals aiming to improve bone density.

3.   **Age-Related Considerations:** As individuals age, their bodies may respond differently to certain types of exercises. Tailoring routines to consider age-related changes in flexibility, muscle mass, and recovery times is crucial. This personalized approach accommodates the specific needs of women over 60, ensuring that exercises align with their life stage.

4.   **Sustainability and Enjoyment**: Fitness is more likely to become a sustainable part of one's lifestyle when routines are enjoyable and aligned with personal preferences. Tailoring routines allows individuals to engage in activities they find pleasurable, increasing the likelihood of adherence to the exercise regimen.

5.   **Comprehensive Fitness**: A well-rounded fitness routine addresses various aspects of physical well-being. Incorporating a mix of aerobic exercises, strength training, flexibility exercises, and balance-enhancing activities ensures a comprehensive approach. Aerobic exercises promote cardiovascular health, strength training supports muscle and bone health, flexibility exercises enhance joint mobility, and balance activities reduce the risk of falls.

6.   **Progression and Adaptation**: Tailoring routines allows for continuous adaptation as individuals progress in their fitness journey. It enables the gradual incorporation of more challenging exercises or adjustments based on improvements in strength, endurance, or overall fitness levels.

In summary, a personalized approach to exercise recognizes the individuality of each person's fitness journey, accounting for health considerations, age-related factors, and personal preferences. By incorporating a mix of exercises that address various aspects of fitness, individuals can create a routine that not only meets their unique needs but also enhances their overall well-being.

Aerobic Exercises

Here's a comprehensive list of aerobic exercises that can be tailored to various fitness levels and preferences:

1. Walking:

   - Brisk walking or power walking
   - Walking on an incline or uphill

2. Running/Jogging:

   - Running at a steady pace
   - Interval running (alternating between high and low intensity)

3. Cycling:

   - Outdoor cycling
   - Stationary cycling or spinning classes

4. Swimming:

   - Lap swimming
   - Water aerobics

5. Jump Rope:

   - Traditional jump rope exercises
   - High-intensity interval jump rope workouts

6. Dancing:

   - Zumba
   - Aerobic dance classes

7. Kickboxing:

   - Aerobic kickboxing routines
   - Kickboxing classes

8. High-Intensity Interval Training (HIIT):

   - Short bursts of intense exercise followed by rest
   - Example: Burpees, jumping jacks, mountain climbers

9. Rowing:

- Rowing machine workouts
- Outdoor rowing
10. Elliptical Training:
- Using an elliptical machine
- Mimicking the motion of running without impact
11. Stair Climbing:
- Climbing stairs at home or using a stair climber machine - Alternating between stepping up and down for variation
12. Aerobic Step Classes:
- Choreographed step routines
- Incorporating a step bench for added intensity
13. Circuit Training:
- Rotating through various aerobic exercises with minimal rest
- Combining strength and aerobic exercises in a circuit
14. Group Fitness Classes:
- Participating in classes like BodyCombat, BodyAttack, or Cardio Sculpt
- Group exercise settings provide motivation and variety
15. Sports Activities:
- Tennis
- Basketball
- Soccer
- Any sport that involves continuous movement

Remember to start at an intensity that suits your fitness level and gradually increase as your endurance improves. Always consult with a healthcare professional before starting a new exercise program, especially if you have any existing health conditions.

Strength Exercises

Here's a comprehensive list of strength training exercises that target various muscle groups. These exercises can be adapted for different fitness levels and preferences:

Upper Body:

1. Push-Ups:

- Standard push-ups
- Incline push-ups for beginners - Decline push-ups for added difficulty

2. Pull-Ups/Chin-Ups:

- Wide grip for back emphasis - Close grip for biceps emphasis

3. Dumbbell Bench Press:

- Flat bench, incline, or decline variations - Alternatives: Barbell bench press, machine chest press

4. Dumbbell Rows: - Bent-over rows

- Single-arm rows

5. Overhead Shoulder Press:

- Dumbbell or barbell variations
- Alternatives: Arnold press, seated shoulder press

6. Bicep Curls:

- Standing or seated curls - Hammer curls for forearm engagement

7. Tricep Dips:

- Using parallel bars or a sturdy surface
- Bench dips for beginners

8. Lateral Raises:

- Lifting arms to the sides to target shoulders
- Front raises for anterior deltoids

Lower Body:

1. Squats:

- Bodyweight squats
- Barbell back squats or front squats
- Sumo squats for inner thighs

2. Deadlifts:

- Conventional deadlifts - Romanian deadlifts for hamstrings

3. Lunges:

- Forward lunges
- Reverse lunges
- Walking lunges for added challenge

4. Leg Press:

- Using a leg press machine - Single-leg press for unilateral work

5. Calf Raises:

- Standing or seated calf raises
- Using a calf raise machine

6. Glute Bridges:

- Standard glute bridges
- Single-leg glute bridges

Core:

1. Planks:

- Front plank
- Side plank
- Plank variations (e.g., plank with shoulder taps)

2. Russian Twists:

- Seated or lying down with a twist
- Using a medicine ball or weight for added resistance

3. Leg Raises:

- Lying down or hanging leg raises
- Flutter kicks for lower abs

4. Woodchoppers:

- Using a cable machine or resistance band
- Engages obliques and core rotation

5. Hollow Body Hold:

- Lying down with arms and legs raised
- Challenges the entire core

Remember to maintain proper form during strength training exercises, and start with a weight that allows for controlled movements. Gradually increase the intensity as your strength improves. If you're new to strength training or have any health concerns, consider consulting with a fitness professional or healthcare provider.

Flexibility Exercises

Here's a comprehensive list of flexibility exercises that can improve your range of motion, reduce muscle stiffness, and enhance overall flexibility. Perform these exercises as part of a warm-up or cool-down routine, and aim to hold each stretch for 15-30 seconds, gradually increasing the duration as your flexibility improves:

Neck and Shoulders:

1. Neck Tilt:

- Gently tilt your head to one side, bringing your ear toward your shoulder. - Repeat on the other side.

2. Neck Rotation:

- Turn your head to one side, looking over your shoulder. - Repeat on the other side.

3. Shoulder Rolls:

- Roll your shoulders forward and backward in circular motions.

4. Shoulder Stretch:

- Bring one arm across your chest and gently press it with the opposite hand. - Repeat on the other side.

Upper Body:

5. Triceps Stretch:

- Reach your hand down your back and gently press on your elbow with the opposite hand.

6. Chest Opener:

- Clasp your hands behind your back and straighten your arms, lifting them slightly.

Back:

7. Cat-Cow Stretch:

- Start on your hands and knees. Arch your back upward (cat) and then lower it while lifting your head (cow).

8. Child's Pose:

- Kneel on the floor, sit back on your heels, and stretch your arms forward.

Lower Body:

9. Hamstring Stretch:

- Sit on the floor with one leg extended and the other foot against the inner thigh. Reach for your toes.

10. Quad Stretch:
- Stand on one leg, bring the opposite foot toward your buttocks, and hold your ankle.
11. Calf Stretch:
- Stand facing a wall, place your hands on it, and step one foot back, keeping it straight. Bend the front knee.
12. Hip Flexor Stretch:
- Step one foot forward into a lunge position, keeping the back leg straight. Sink into the stretch.

Hips and Glutes:

13. Pigeon Pose:
- From a plank position, bring one knee toward the same-side wrist and extend the other leg straight behind you.
14. Butterfly Stretch:
- Sit with the soles of your feet together and gently press your knees toward the floor.

Legs and Ankles:

15. Ankle Circles:
- Lift one foot and rotate your ankle in circular motions.
16. Seated Forward Bend:
- Sit with your legs extended, hinge at your hips, and reach toward your toes.

Remember to perform these flexibility exercises regularly to maintain and improve flexibility over time. If you have any existing health conditions or concerns, consult with a healthcare provider or fitness professional before starting a new flexibility routine.

Balance Enhancing Activities

Here's a comprehensive list of balance-enhancing activities that help improve stability, coordination, and proprioception. Incorporating these activities into your routine can contribute to overall balance and reduce the risk of falls. Start with activities that match your current fitness level and gradually progress as your balance improves:

1. Single-Leg Stands:

- Stand on one leg for 15-30 seconds, then switch to the other leg.
- Progress by closing your eyes or incorporating head turns.

2. Heel-to-Toe Walk:

- Walk in a straight line, placing the heel of one foot directly in front of the toes of the other.
- Focus on maintaining a straight line and steady pace.

3. Balancing on a BOSU Ball:

- Stand on a BOSU ball with the dome side down for added instability. - Progress to single-leg stands on the BOSU.

4. Tai Chi:

- This martial art emphasizes slow, controlled movements that enhance balance and flexibility.
- Attend a Tai Chi class or follow online tutorials.

5. Yoga Poses:

- Tree Pose: Stand on one leg and place the sole of the other foot against the inner thigh or calf.
- Warrior III: Balance on one leg while extending the other leg and torso parallel to the ground.

6. Stability Ball Exercises:

- Perform exercises like seated marches or seated balances on a stability ball. - Gradually progress to standing on the stability ball.

7. Walking on Uneven Surfaces:

- Walk on grass, sand, or cobblestone paths to challenge your balance. - Use caution and start with stable surfaces before advancing.

8. Tandem Walk:

- Walk in a straight line, placing the heel of one foot directly in front of the toes of the other.
- Progress by turning your head or closing your eyes.

9. Standing Leg Swings:

- Hold onto a support and swing one leg forward and backward. - Gradually increase the height and speed of the swings.

10. Dynamic Balance Exercises:

- Side leg lifts: Lift one leg to the side while maintaining balance.
- Clock reaches: Stand on one leg and reach your other foot forward, to the side, and behind you in a clock-like motion.

11. Balance Board Exercises:

- Use a balance board to perform exercises like rocking side to side or front to back.
- Progress to standing on one leg on the balance board.

12. Functional Movements:

- Practice activities that mimic daily movements, such as rising from a chair or reaching for items on a shelf.
- Focus on controlled, deliberate movements.

Incorporate these activities into your routine regularly to enhance your balance and stability. If you have any existing health conditions or concerns, consult with a healthcare provider or fitness professional before starting a new balance-enhancing routine.

Symbiotic Relationship between Exercise and Keto

The symbiotic relationship between exercise and the keto diet is crucial for several reasons, contributing to overall health and well-being. Here are key aspects of this relationship:

1. Enhanced Fat Utilization:

- The keto diet emphasizes a low-carbohydrate intake, leading the body to enter a state of ketosis. In ketosis, the body becomes efficient at burning fats for energy instead of relying on carbohydrates.
- Regular exercise complements this process by further enhancing the body's ability to utilize stored fats for energy. This synergy promotes more effective fat loss and weight management.

2. Improved Metabolic Health:

- Both the keto diet and exercise independently contribute to improved metabolic health. The combination can have synergistic effects, enhancing insulin sensitivity and supporting better blood sugar control.
- Exercise helps muscle cells become more receptive to insulin, promoting efficient glucose uptake and reducing the risk of insulin resistance.

3. Preservation of Lean Muscle Mass:

- The keto diet, when combined with adequate protein intake, can support the preservation of lean muscle mass during weight loss. This is essential for maintaining strength, functionality, and metabolic rate.
- Resistance training or strength exercises further promote muscle preservation and development.

4. Increased Endurance and Stamina:

- As the body adapts to the keto diet, endurance athletes may experience improved performance. The reliance on fat as a primary fuel source can enhance endurance and stamina during prolonged exercise.
- Engaging in regular aerobic exercise, such as running or cycling, can further optimize cardiovascular health and endurance on the keto diet.

5. Positive Impact on Mental Health:

- Both the keto diet and exercise have been linked to positive effects on mental health. The release of endorphins during exercise contributes to mood enhancement and stress reduction.

\-   The neuroprotective properties of ketones produced during ketosis may also have cognitive benefits, potentially supporting mental clarity and focus.

6. Efficient Recovery:

\-   Adequate protein intake on the keto diet supports muscle repair and recovery after exercise. Essential amino acids from protein are crucial for rebuilding tissues and promoting recovery.
\-   Incorporating post-exercise meals that align with keto principles helps replenish glycogen stores and optimize recovery.

7. Holistic Approach to Health:

- Combining the keto diet with regular exercise creates a holistic approach to health. The diet addresses nutritional aspects, optimizing fuel sources, while exercise promotes cardiovascular health, strength, flexibility, and overall fitness.

8. Weight Management and Long-Term Health:

- The synergistic effect of the keto diet and exercise contributes to sustainable weight management. This combination has the potential to support long-term health by addressing multiple facets of well-being.

In summary, the symbiotic relationship between the keto diet and exercise offers a comprehensive approach to health, encompassing metabolic optimization, physical fitness, mental well-being, and long-term vitality. Individual responses may vary, so it's advisable to consult with healthcare and fitness professionals to tailor the approach to personal goals and health conditions.

CHAPTER10:HOWTOLOSEWEIGHT AND KEEP IT OFF

Losing weight is a journey that extends beyond shedding pounds; it's about adopting sustainable habits that promote long-term health and well-being. In this chapter, we delve into strategies for sustainable weight loss and offer tips for maintaining your weight loss success while embracing a healthy lifestyle.

1. Crafting Sustainable Habits:

Sustainable weight loss begins with the cultivation of healthy habits. Let's explore the importance of gradual changes, emphasizing consistency over drastic measures. Adopting sustainable habits ensures that weight loss is not only achievable but also maintainable in the long run.

Sustainable weight loss is a journey guided by the cultivation of healthy habits, and its foundation lies in the deliberate embrace of gradual changes. The emphasis here is not on rapid transformations or drastic measures but on the steady integration of behaviors that promote a healthier lifestyle. The importance of this approach is multifaceted, contributing significantly to the achievability and maintainability of weight loss in the long run.

Gradual Changes for Lasting Impact:

Making gradual changes allows individuals to adapt to new habits at a pace that aligns with their lifestyle and preferences. This approach acknowledges that sustainable weight loss is not an overnight accomplishment but a series of small, meaningful adjustments over time. By gradually introducing changes, individuals are more likely to incorporate them into their daily routines, fostering a sense of normalcy and reducing the likelihood of resistance or burnout.

Consistency Over Drastic Measures:

Consistency is the cornerstone of sustainable weight loss. While drastic measures may yield rapid results initially, they often prove challenging to maintain over the long term. By focusing on consistent, sustainable habits, individuals build a foundation for lasting success. This involves creating a lifestyle that aligns with their values, preferences, and overall well-being.

Behavioral Shifts and Lifestyle Integration:

Sustainable weight loss is not solely about what one eats but also about how one lives. Gradual changes allow for the integration of new behaviors into daily life seamlessly. This might involve incorporating physical activity, developing mindful eating practices, and adopting a more positive relationship with food. As these behaviors become ingrained in one's lifestyle, they contribute to a sustainable and holistic approach to weight management.

Cultivating Healthy Habits for Life:

The beauty of cultivating healthy habits lies in their potential to extend beyond weight loss goals. These habits become integral parts of a person's identity and contribute to overall well-being. Whether it's choosing nutrient-dense foods, staying physically active, or prioritizing self-care, these habits form the building blocks of a healthy and fulfilling life.

Long-Term Maintenance and Lifestyle Harmony:

Sustainable habits pave the way for weight loss maintenance by creating a lifestyle that individuals find enjoyable and sustainable. This harmony between habits and lifestyle means that individuals are more likely to stick with their healthier choices, preventing the cycle of yo-yo dieting often associated with drastic measures.

In essence, the journey toward sustainable weight loss is a marathon, not a sprint. By embracing gradual changes and prioritizing consistency, individuals not only achieve their weight loss goals but also lay the groundwork for a healthier, more fulfilling life in the long run. This approach fosters resilience, adaptability, and a sense of empowerment, making the quest for well-being an enduring and rewarding endeavor.

2. Nutrient-Dense Eating:

We cannot stress enough the significance of nutrient-dense foods in supporting weight loss and overall health. Let's learn how to build meals that prioritize essential nutrients, providing your body with the fuel it needs while managing calorie intake. A focus on whole, unprocessed foods becomes a cornerstone of lasting weight management.

Building meals that prioritize essential nutrients while managing calorie intake involves a thoughtful approach to food selection and portion control. Here's a guide on creating nutrient-dense meals and why a focus on whole, unprocessed foods is crucial for lasting weight management:

1. Choose a Colorful Plate:

- Aim for a diverse range of colorful vegetables and fruits to ensure a spectrum of vitamins, minerals, and antioxidants. Different colors often indicate varying nutrient profiles, so incorporating a rainbow of produce contributes to overall nutrient density.

2. Prioritize Lean Proteins:

- Include lean protein sources like poultry, fish, tofu, legumes, and lean cuts of meat. Protein is essential for muscle maintenance, satiety, and overall metabolic health. Opt for grilled, baked, or steamed preparations to keep the meal lean.

3. Include Whole Grains:

- Opt for whole grains such as quinoa, brown rice, oats, or whole wheat. These grains offer fiber, vitamins, and minerals, providing sustained energy and promoting digestive health. Whole grains also contribute to a feeling of fullness, aiding in managing calorie intake.

4. Incorporate Healthy Fats:

- Choose sources of healthy fats, such as avocados, nuts, seeds, and olive oil. Healthy fats are crucial for nutrient absorption and satiety. While fats are energydense, their inclusion in moderate amounts contributes to a satisfying and wellbalanced meal.

5. Watch Portion Sizes:

- Be mindful of portion sizes to manage calorie intake effectively. Use smaller plates and bowls, and listen to your body's hunger and fullness cues. Understanding appropriate portion sizes ensures you enjoy your meal while staying within your caloric goals.

6. Minimize Processed Foods:

- Processed foods often contain added sugars, unhealthy fats, and excess sodium. Minimize the intake of pre-packaged and processed items. Instead, focus on whole, unprocessed foods to provide your body with the essential nutrients it needs without unnecessary additives.

7. Hydrate with Water:

- Water is a vital component of a nutrient-dense meal. Stay hydrated by choosing water as your primary beverage. Avoid sugary drinks and excessive amounts of caffeinated beverages, as they can contribute unnecessary calories and potentially disrupt nutrient absorption.

8. Plan Balanced Meals:

- Plan meals that include a balance of macronutrients—proteins, carbohydrates, and fats. This balance ensures sustained energy, supports metabolic functions, and prevents nutrient deficiencies. Consider consulting with a nutritionist for personalized guidance based on your specific needs.

9. Be Mindful of Snacking:

- If snacking is part of your routine, choose nutrient-dense snacks like fresh fruit, vegetables with hummus, or a handful of nuts. Mindful snacking can contribute to overall nutrient intake without derailing your weight management goals.

10. Enjoy Whole, Unprocessed Foods:

- Whole, unprocessed foods provide the body with a wide array of essential nutrients in their natural state. These foods are rich in fiber, vitamins, and minerals, offering optimal nutrition while supporting lasting weight management.

In summary, building meals that prioritize essential nutrients involves a well-rounded selection of colorful, whole, unprocessed foods. This approach not only supports weight loss goals by managing calorie intake but also promotes overall health and well-being. By embracing nutrient-dense choices, you create a sustainable foundation for lasting weight management and a healthier lifestyle.

3. Mindful Eating Practices:

Now let's explore the concept of mindful eating and its role in weight management. By cultivating awareness around hunger, fullness, and the eating experience, you'll develop a healthier relationship with food. Mindful eating practices contribute to a more intuitive approach to nourishment, aiding in weight loss sustainability.

Mindful eating is a transformative approach that can profoundly impact weight management by fostering a healthier relationship with food. By cultivating awareness around hunger, fullness, and the overall eating experience, individuals develop a more intuitive approach to nourishment, contributing to weight loss sustainability.

1. Cultivating Awareness:

- Mindful eating encourages individuals to be fully present during meals. It involves paying attention to the sensory aspects of eating, such as the flavors, textures, and aromas of food. By becoming more aware of these elements, one develops a deeper connection with the act of eating.

2. Recognizing Hunger and Fullness:

- Mindful eating prompts individuals to tune in to their body's hunger and fullness cues. This awareness helps distinguish between physical hunger and emotional or external triggers for eating. By responding to genuine hunger and stopping when comfortably full, individuals naturally regulate their caloric intake.

3. Eating with Intention:

- Mindful eating emphasizes the importance of intentionality in food choices. It encourages individuals to choose foods that provide both nourishment and satisfaction. This intentional approach to eating helps prevent mindless snacking or overindulgence in response to external cues.

4. Slowing Down the Eating Pace:

- Mindful eating advocates for savoring each bite and slowing down the eating pace. This intentional slowing allows the body's natural satiety signals to catch up with food consumption, preventing overeating. Enjoying the process of eating contributes to a more fulfilling and satisfying meal experience.

5. Emotional Connection to Food:

- Many individuals have complex emotional relationships with food. Mindful eating prompts reflection on emotional triggers for eating, helping individuals understand and address emotional eating patterns. This self-awareness is crucial for sustainable weight management.

6. Reducing Stress-Related Eating:

- Stress can influence eating behaviors. Mindful eating practices, such as deep breathing or mindful pauses before meals, contribute to stress reduction. By managing stress, individuals are less likely to turn to food as a coping mechanism, supporting weight loss goals.

7. Developing Intuitive Eating:

- Mindful eating is closely linked to intuitive eating—a philosophy that encourages individuals to trust their body's natural cues for hunger, fullness, and food preferences. This intuitive approach fosters a sustainable and flexible relationship with food, enhancing weight loss sustainability.

8. Enhancing Self-Regulation:

- Mindful eating empowers individuals to become more attuned to their body's needs. This heightened self-awareness supports self-regulation, helping individuals make mindful choices about portion sizes, food quality, and overall dietary patterns.

9. Mindful Eating Practices:

- Incorporating practices such as mindful breathing, pausing before eating, and recognizing the impact of distractions during meals enhances the overall mindful eating experience. These practices contribute to a more positive relationship with food and support weight management efforts.

10. Long-Term Weight Management:

- By developing mindfulness around eating habits, individuals lay the foundation for sustainable weight management. Mindful eating practices contribute to a more balanced, enjoyable, and intentional approach to nourishment, aligning with longterm health and wellness goals.

In summary, mindful eating is a powerful tool in weight management, emphasizing awareness, intentionality, and the development of an intuitive connection with food. By fostering a mindful approach to eating, individuals can cultivate a healthier relationship with food, leading to sustainable and lasting weight loss.

4. Physical Activity for Weight Maintenance:

Regular physical activity is not just a tool for weight loss but a key component of weight maintenance. Let's discover how incorporating exercise into your routine supports calorie expenditure, enhances metabolism, and contributes to overall wellbeing. We provide practical tips for staying active in the long term.

Incorporating regular exercise into your routine is a key factor in supporting calorie expenditure, enhancing metabolism, and contributing to overall well-being. Here's a brief overview:

1. Calorie Expenditure:

- Exercise increases the number of calories your body burns, aiding in weight management. Both aerobic exercises (like walking or jogging) and strength training contribute to calorie expenditure. The more intense the activity, the more calories you burn during and after the workout.

2. Metabolism Boost:

- Regular physical activity boosts your metabolism, helping your body efficiently process and utilize calories. This effect continues even after you've finished exercising, contributing to long-term metabolic health. Strength training, in particular, helps build lean muscle, which further supports a higher resting metabolic rate.

3. Cardiovascular Health:

- Aerobic exercises, such as cycling or swimming, enhance cardiovascular health by improving heart and lung function. This not only contributes to overall well-being but also supports efficient oxygen transport and nutrient delivery throughout the body.

4. Mental and Emotional Benefits:

- Exercise has proven mental health benefits, reducing stress, anxiety, and depression. Physical activity stimulates the release of endorphins, promoting a positive mood and enhancing overall well-being. Establishing a routine that includes exercise can contribute to improved mental resilience.

5. Increased Energy Levels:

- Contrary to the misconception that exercise depletes energy, regular physical activity actually increases energy levels. It improves circulation and oxygen flow, making you feel more alert and energized throughout the day.

6. Better Sleep:

- Quality sleep is essential for overall health, and exercise plays a role in promoting better sleep patterns. Engaging in physical activity can help regulate sleep cycles, leading to more restful and rejuvenating sleep.

7. Long-Term Habit Formation:

- To make exercise sustainable, choose activities you enjoy. Whether it's walking, dancing, or participating in a team sport, finding activities that bring pleasure increases the likelihood of sticking to your routine over the long term.

8. Consistency Is Key:

- Consistency is crucial for reaping the benefits of exercise. Rather than focusing on intense, sporadic workouts, aim for regular, moderate activity. This approach not only enhances overall fitness but also establishes a sustainable routine.

9. Set Realistic Goals:

- Set achievable and realistic goals based on your fitness level. Gradual progress is more sustainable than attempting drastic changes. Celebrate small victories, and adjust your goals as you build strength and endurance.

10. Mix It Up:

- Prevent boredom by incorporating variety into your exercise routine. This can include a mix of cardiovascular exercises, strength training, flexibility exercises, and activities you genuinely enjoy. Variety not only keeps things interesting but also engages different muscle groups for a well-rounded fitness approach.

In summary, incorporating exercise into your routine supports calorie expenditure, boosts metabolism, and contributes to overall well-being. The key is to find activities you enjoy, set realistic goals, and maintain consistency for long-term benefits. By making exercise a regular part of your lifestyle, you promote not only physical health but also mental and emotional wellness.

5. Behavioral Strategies for Weight Maintenance:

Behavioral strategies play a crucial role in maintaining weight loss. Let's uncover techniques to navigate challenges, manage stress, and build resilience against setbacks. We'll explore the psychological aspects of weight maintenance, empowering you to overcome obstacles on your journey.

Navigating challenges, managing stress, and building resilience are integral components of a successful weight maintenance journey. Here are some techniques to address these aspects:

1. Mindful Stress Management:

- Incorporate stress-management techniques into your daily routine. This may include mindfulness meditation, deep breathing exercises, or yoga. These practices can help reduce stress levels, fostering a healthier mindset and minimizing the likelihood of stress-induced eating.

2. Goal Reframing:

- Embrace a mindset of continuous improvement. Instead of viewing setbacks as failures, consider them opportunities to learn and adjust your approach. Reframe your goals into positive, achievable steps, allowing for flexibility in your weight maintenance journey.

3. Social Support:

- Cultivate a support system of friends, family, or fellow individuals on a similar journey. Sharing experiences, challenges, and successes with others can provide encouragement and a sense of camaraderie, making it easier to navigate obstacles.

4. Establishing Routine:

- Create a structured routine that includes regular meals, exercise, and self-care. Having a consistent daily schedule provides stability and reduces decision fatigue, making it easier to adhere to healthy habits.

5. Identifying Triggers:

- Recognize emotional triggers that may lead to overeating or unhealthy habits. This self-awareness allows you to develop alternative coping mechanisms, such as engaging in a hobby, going for a walk, or practicing relaxation techniques.

6. Celebrate Non-Scale Victories:

- Shift the focus from solely scale-related achievements to non-scale victories. Acknowledge and celebrate improvements in energy levels, mood, fitness achievements, or other positive changes in your overall well-being.

7. Professional Support:

- Consider seeking guidance from a healthcare professional, nutritionist, or mental health counselor. They can provide personalized advice, strategies, and support tailored to your specific challenges and goals.

8. Regular Reflection:

- Set aside time for regular self-reflection. Evaluate your progress, identify areas for improvement, and celebrate your successes. This practice fosters self-awareness and helps you stay committed to your long-term goals.

9. Resilience Building:

- Understand that setbacks are a natural part of any journey. Building resilience involves developing the ability to bounce back from challenges. Learn from experiences, adapt, and stay focused on your commitment to a healthy lifestyle.

10. Adaptive Mindset:

- Embrace an adaptive mindset that welcomes change and sees challenges as opportunities for growth. This mindset shift can empower you to navigate the ups and downs of weight maintenance with resilience and determination.

In summary, managing stress, building resilience, and navigating challenges in weight maintenance involve adopting a holistic approach that addresses both physical and psychological aspects. By integrating these techniques into your daily life, you can create a sustainable and resilient foundation for maintaining a healthy weight.

6. Balancing Macros for Maintenance:

Maintaining a balanced macronutrient intake is essential for sustaining weight loss. Let's discuss how to adapt your macronutrient ratios as you transition from active weight loss to maintenance. This ensures that you continue to fuel your body optimally while preventing weight regain.

As you transition from active weight loss to maintenance, adapting your macronutrient ratios is crucial to sustain your progress. Here's a brief guide on how to approach this transition:

1. Gradual Adjustments:

- Instead of making abrupt changes, consider adjusting your macronutrient ratios gradually. Small, incremental adjustments allow your body to adapt without causing significant disruptions.

2. Monitoring Progress:

- Regularly assess your progress and how your body responds to the current macronutrient ratios. Pay attention to energy levels, satiety, and overall well-being. This feedback will guide you in making informed adjustments.

3. Assessing Caloric Needs:

- Determine your maintenance caloric needs based on factors like age, activity level, and metabolism. Calculate the caloric intake required to maintain your current weight and adjust macronutrient ratios accordingly.

4. Protein Intake:

- Maintain a sufficient protein intake to support muscle preservation and overall health. Protein plays a crucial role in body composition and satiety, contributing to a balanced macronutrient profile.

5. Adjusting Fat and Carbohydrates:

- Depending on your preferences and individual response, you can make adjustments to the ratios of fats and carbohydrates. Some individuals may thrive on a higher fat intake, while others may find a balanced approach with moderate carbohydrates more suitable.

6. Listen to Your Body:

- Tune in to your body's signals and adjust macronutrient ratios based on hunger, energy levels, and performance during physical activities. This intuitive approach helps you find a sustainable balance that aligns with your lifestyle.

7. Periodic Assessments:

- Periodically reassess your macronutrient ratios, especially if you experience changes in physical activity, lifestyle, or health status. Your dietary needs may evolve over time, requiring adjustments for long-term sustainability.

8. Professional Guidance:

- If needed, consult with a healthcare professional or nutritionist for personalized advice. They can provide insights based on your individual health goals, metabolic rate, and dietary preferences.

9. Lifestyle Considerations:

- Consider your overall lifestyle, including stress levels, sleep quality, and daily activities. These factors can influence how your body responds to different macronutrient ratios, guiding your adjustments.

10. Sustainable Choices:

- Emphasize sustainability in your dietary choices. Opt for nutrient-dense, whole foods that contribute to your overall well-being. This approach ensures that your macronutrient ratios support both your health goals and a lasting, balanced lifestyle.

In summary, adapting macronutrient ratios during the transition from active weight loss to maintenance involves a personalized and gradual approach. By monitoring your body's signals, making informed adjustments, and prioritizing sustainable choices, you can establish a macronutrient profile that supports your long-term health and wellness.

7. Setting Realistic Goals:

Realistic goal-setting is fundamental to long-term success. We'll guide you through the process of establishing achievable objectives that align with your individual health aspirations. The focus is on gradual, sustainable progress rather than rapid, short-term changes.

Establishing achievable objectives aligned with your individual health aspirations involves a thoughtful and realistic approach. Here's a brief guide to help you through this process:

1. Reflect on Your Goals:

- Begin by reflecting on your health aspirations. Identify specific areas you want to improve, whether it's weight management, energy levels, or overall well-being. Having clear goals provides direction for your objectives.

2. Break Down Larger Goals:

- If you have broad health goals, break them down into smaller, more manageable objectives. For example, if weight loss is a goal, consider setting monthly targets to make progress more achievable.

3. Prioritize Objectives:

- Prioritize your objectives based on their significance and impact on your overall well-being. This helps you focus on the most critical aspects of your health and prevents overwhelm.

4. Be Realistic:

- Set realistic and attainable objectives. Consider your current lifestyle, commitments, and potential challenges. Setting goals that are too ambitious can lead to frustration, while realistic objectives are more likely to be sustained.

5. Define Actionable Steps:

- Outline specific, actionable steps to achieve each objective. Break down the process into smaller tasks that you can integrate into your daily routine. These steps should be practical and fit seamlessly into your lifestyle.

6. Consider a Timeline:

- Establish a timeline for your objectives. Determine reasonable timeframes for achieving each goal, keeping in mind that some objectives may require more time than others. A timeline provides structure and accountability.

7. Track Progress:

- Regularly monitor your progress. Keep a journal, use apps, or create a system that allows you to track your achievements. Celebrate small victories along the way to stay motivated.

8. Adjust as Needed:

- Be flexible and willing to adjust your objectives based on your evolving needs and circumstances. Life is dynamic, and adapting your goals ensures continued progress.

9. Seek Support:

- Share your objectives with friends, family, or a supportive community. Having a network that encourages and understands your health journey can provide valuable support and motivation.

10. Celebrate Achievements:

- Celebrate your achievements, no matter how small. Acknowledge the positive changes you've made and the progress you've achieved. Celebrating success reinforces your commitment to your health journey.

Remember, the key to establishing achievable objectives is to approach the process with self-compassion, patience, and a commitment to long-term well-being. By setting realistic goals, defining actionable steps, and staying adaptable, you can create a roadmap that guides you toward your individual health aspirations.

8. Cultivating a Supportive Environment:

Your environment plays a significant role in your ability to maintain weight loss. Learn how to create a supportive living space that encourages healthy choices. We'll discuss the impact of social support and offer guidance on building a network that fosters your weight management goals.

Creating a supportive living space that encourages healthy choices involves thoughtful adjustments to your environment. Here's a brief guide to help you foster a setting conducive to well-being:

1. Organize for Accessibility:

- Arrange healthy food options prominently in your kitchen. Make fruits, vegetables, and nutritious snacks easily accessible, while placing less healthy choices out of immediate sight.

2. Meal Prep Convenience:

- Simplify healthy eating by prepping meals and snacks in advance. Store pre-cut fruits, veggies, and portioned meals in your refrigerator for quick and convenient choices.

3. Hydration Station:

- Keep water readily available and visible. Place water bottles or a pitcher with fresh lemon or cucumber slices on your kitchen counter or workspace to encourage regular hydration.

4. Create a Workout Zone:

- Designate a space for exercise at home. Whether it's a small corner for yoga or a dedicated home gym, having a designated workout zone can motivate you to stay active.

5. Mindful Eating Environment:

- Establish a designated eating area free from distractions like TV or screens. Creating a mindful environment during meals can promote conscious eating habits and prevent overconsumption.

6. Natural Light and Greenery:

- Open curtains and let in natural light to boost mood and energy levels.

Incorporate indoor plants to improve air quality and create a calming atmosphere.

7. Declutter for Mental Clarity:

- Decluttering your living space can positively impact your mental well-being. A tidy environment can reduce stress and create a sense of order, making it easier to focus on healthy choices.

8. Limit Unhealthy Snacks:

- Minimize the presence of sugary or processed snacks in your home. If they're not readily available, you're less likely to indulge in unhealthy choices.

9. Incorporate Visual Reminders:

- Use visual cues to remind yourself of your health goals. This could include positive affirmations, motivational quotes, or images that inspire you to make healthier choices.

10. Family and Community Support:

- Involve your family or housemates in creating a health-conscious environment. Shared goals and mutual support can enhance the positive impact of your living space on everyone's well-being.

By making intentional adjustments to your living space, you can create an environment that supports your health and wellness goals. These simple changes can have a profound effect on your lifestyle choices and contribute to a positive, healthfocused atmosphere at home.

By understanding the interplay of habits, nutrition, exercise, and mindset, you'll be equipped with the tools needed to not only achieve weight loss but to sustain it for a lifetime.

CONCLUSION

As we wrap up this journey through "Keto Diet for Women Over 60," let's recap the key takeaways that can empower you on your keto journey:

1. Tailored Guidance:

- This book provides personalized advice crafted for the unique needs and aspirations of women aged 60 and above embarking on a keto lifestyle.

2. Holistic Approach:

- Beyond weight loss, the keto diet offers a holistic strategy for enhancing overall well-being. It addresses age-related health concerns, supports sustainable weight management, and promotes vitality.

3. Practical Tools:

- Find practical tools, evidence-based insights, and actionable advice to guide you on your keto journey. From meal planning to overcoming challenges, the book equips you with the resources needed for success.

4. Healthy Aging:

- Embrace the physiological changes that accompany aging by understanding how keto can be a game-changer. It's not just a diet; it's a lifestyle fostering improved health and longevity.

Encouragement for Your Journey:

- Your keto journey is a step toward a more vibrant and healthier life. The commitment you've shown to your well-being is commendable. Remember, progress is a journey, not a destination.

Continuing Your Keto Path:

- Stay connected to the keto community for ongoing support and inspiration. Share your experiences, seek advice, and celebrate victories. Consistency and a positive mindset will propel you toward your health goals.

Resources for Further Information:

- To deepen your understanding and find additional support, explore reputable sources and communities. Reliable websites, nutritionists, and local keto groups can provide valuable insights tailored to your needs.

Acknowledging Your Journey:

- Celebrate your achievements, both big and small. Every positive choice is a step toward a healthier, more fulfilling life. The journey doesn't end here—it evolves with each mindful decision you make.

As you continue on your keto journey, remember that you're not alone. The resilience you've shown in seeking a healthier lifestyle is commendable. May this book serve as a steadfast companion on your path to improved well-being. Wishing you success, fulfillment, and vibrant health in the chapters that follow. Keep thriving!

Don't forget to scan the QR Code to get all bonus content!